Viral Haemorrhagic Fevers

PERSPECTIVES IN MEDICAL VIROLOGY

Volume 11

Series Editors

A.J. Zuckerman

Royal Free and University College Medical School
University College London
London, UK

I.K. Mushahwar

Abbott Laboratories
Viral Discovery Group
Abbott Park, IL, USA

Viral Haemorrhagic Fevers

Colin R. Howard

Royal Veterinary College
Royal College Street
London NW1 0TU
United Kingdom

2005

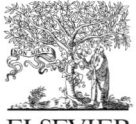

ELSEVIER

Amsterdam – Boston – Heidelberg – London – New York – Oxford
Paris – San Diego – San Francisco – Singapore – Sydney – Tokyo

ELSEVIER B.V.
Sara Burgerhartstraat 25
P.O. Box 211, 1000 AE Amsterdam
The Netherlands

ELSEVIER Inc.
525 B Street, Suite 1900
San Diego, CA 92101-4495
USA

ELSEVIER Ltd
The Boulevard, Langford Lane
Kidlington, Oxford OX5 1GB
UK

ELSEVIER Ltd
84 Theobalds Road
London WC1X 8RR
UK

1st edition 2005

Library of Congress Cataloging in Publication Data
A catalog record is available from the Library of Congress.

British Library Cataloguing in Publication Data
A catalogue record is available from the British Library.

ISBN: 0-444-50660-8
ISSN: 0168-7069

⊗ The paper used in this publication meets the requirements of ANSI/NISO Z39.48-1992 (Permanence of Paper).
Printed in The Netherlands.

To Ron Howard
(1922–2003)

Contents

viii

Preface

Infectious disease continues to have a profound effect on society, the economic development of nations, how we relate to the environment around us and with the animals with which we share this planet. Despite the ever increasing technology that surrounds us in our daily lives, few of us escape the ravages and aftermaths of infectious disease, whether it be something as relatively discomforting as the common cold or more serious such as influenza among the elderly or respiratory infections of the newborn. As I complete this monograph yet another new agent has just emerged, that of Severe Acute Respiratory Syndrome (SARS). Due to a hitherto unrecognised coronavirus, this disease caught public health officials completely by surprise. On a lesser scale, but potentially equally threatening, newer agents such as Hendra and Nipah have emerged. Europe and North America have not escaped—West Nile Virus has extended both its range and pathogenic potential since 1999 where previously it was absent. The United Kingdom livestock industry has suffered two blows in less than a decade. First Bovine Spongiform Encephalopathy, and then in 2002 a disastrous re-introduction of foot and mouth virus.

So why write a volume focusing on Viral Haemorrhagic Fevers? The answer lies partly in informing the reader of progress in research and our understanding of these agents against a backdrop of continuing fear these viruses engender among health care workers and the public alike. But also in part because of the resurgence of interest in these diseases, especially given the alarming increase in the numbers of emerging infections now confronting medical and veterinary science. There is much to be learnt from the study of these agents that is directly applicable to other emerging diseases, particularly in relation to how containing these outbreaks requires a high degree of collaboration between different specialists, often working in suboptimal conditions without strong political support and with barely adequate resources.

This book is primarily aimed at health care workers, clinicians and microbiologists wishing to gain a rapid overview as to the nature of these widely varying agents linked only by their propensity of causing serious human disease. The study of viral haemorrhagic fevers is more than just science. It is a story often played out by scientists against a backdrop of poor funding, political unrest and the fear of the unknown. Accounts of bravery and personal sacrifice are frequently intertwined with the more impersonal scientific descriptions of how these agents have come to our attention. They show graphically that we are heavily reliant on a comparatively few dedicated clinicians schooled in the rapidly shrinking discipline of clinical tropical medicine around the world to form the thin blue line of defence against infections. But I also hope that this book will appeal to a wider audience: members of the public, politicians and funding agencies that shape the way society thinks and reacts to infectious disease. There is growing tendency for society to distrust its academic scientists and ascribe failings to them whenever public health measures break down or some adverse event becomes apparent in a few whilst attempting to protect the many. Yet it is those few individuals that society is dependent upon to guard against further incursions by providing the wherewithal for developing robust technologies, reagents and therapies that are presently lacking. It has become unfashionable over the last decades to support research into these viruses, yet it is this skill base society will depend upon in the future to deal with threats from bioterrorists, emergence of new diseases, and the heightened virulence of those previously recognised. Viral haemorrhagic fever research has gone under-supported for decades although this is beginning to change somewhat in the aftermath of the terrorist attacks of September 11th 2001.

There are many that I am indebted to for encouraging my interest in these viruses, but particularly I should like to thank David Simpson. Together with the late Ernie Bowen, David brimmed with energy, enthusiasm and good humour, even in the darkest of times and taught me the importance of perspective when dealing with difficult and dangerous pathogens. I would also thank David Ellis, an electron microscopist *par excellence*. To numerous to mention, my graduate students have been a joy and inspiration, many of whom I am now privileged to count amongst my friends. Also my thanks go out to my long term friends and colleagues Michael Buchmeier and Michael Oldstone in La Jolla who have shown unfailing hospitality on my frequent visits to invigorating California. Above all, I'm forever in the debt of my wife Liane, who together with our daughters have had to endure my constant preoccupation with all things virological over what is now a lifetime.

Colin Howard,
London,
April 2004.

Introduction

The viral haemorrhagic fevers—often included in the wider category of emerging viruses—constantly surprise, both in terms of where they emerge and the sudden severity with which they may strike. Traditionally, viral haemorrhagic fevers were associated with severe human outbreaks that afflicted comparatively few individuals despite causing widespread alarm and the diversion of scarce public health resources. Marburg virus, for example, was first discovered in 1967 and nearly 40 years on the cumulative number of cases has yet to exceed a thousand. Otherwise viral haemorrhagic fevers remained the preserve of those infectious disease specialists with a particular interest in tropical diseases, rarely emerging into the consciousness of clinicians in North America and Europe apart from occasional imported cases. All this changed with the growing awareness that agents of viral haemorrhagic disease along with other geographically restricted agents of severe human disease were evolving into new ecological niches, particularly in periods of abnormal weather and climatic change. A perfect example is the hantaviruses. Although known for many years, interest in the prototype, Hantaan virus, was largely restricted to those with a somewhat esoteric interest in Korean haemorrhagic fever and occasional cases of nephropathia epidemica in Northern Europe, The Balkans and Scandinavia. Then in 1993, with the sudden emergence of an acute respiratory syndrome[1] in the Four Corners region[2] of the United States caused by what is now referred to as the Sin Nombre Virus, these agents were no longer obscure pathogens in the eyes of western clinicians, but major threats to public health. Mobilisation of resources and a refocusing of effort have shown hantaviruses as widespread throughout the Americas. A particularly severe strain was isolated from Argentina by scientists more familiar with identifying and treating Argentine haemorrhagic fever (AHF), a discovery almost certainly dependent upon the heightened awareness of emerging disease among the clinicians involved.

Interest in these agents has been heightened still further by concern among Western governments that at least some of these viruses have the potential to be used as agents of bioterrorism. Although an international consensus had been achieved in the 1960s as to the anathema of biological weapons and the threat they could pose to mankind outside of any theatre of war, we know that clandestine attempts to weaponise haemorrhagic fever viruses continued until the collapse of the Soviet Union. It is debatable whether such efforts continue in regions where political extremism abounds, but the eventuality is taken seriously by those responsible for securing societies from such threats. This in turn

---

[1] Now known as Hantavirus pulmonary syndrome (HPS).
[2] The region bordering the US states of New Mexico, Arizona, Colorado and Utah.

has meant an upsurge of interest in these viruses, with research and development into the causes and prevention of haemorrhagic fevers undergoing somewhat of a renaissance as part of the wider context of monitoring for abnormal disease patterns among societies of the economically developed world. This follows several decades where research into these viruses has been at low ebb. A cursory examination of papers listed in the National Library of Medicine PubMed database shows a steady increase in the volume of dengue research since the mid-1990s (Table 1), a reflection of the growing importance of this virus as a cause of morbidity in ever increasing number of countries, especially in Asia and the tropics. Despite the uplift in research on viral haemorrhagic fevers, the research capacity is still low as judged on research reported in the international literature. For example, despite the growing awareness of hantavirus infections as causing severe respiratory disease in the Americas, the number of papers is barely above 100 per year. This contrasts with, for example, around 780 papers per year on herpes simplex virus (Fig. 1).

Table 1

Viral haemorrhagic fevers: overview and global distribution

Family	Disease	Virus	Vector	Distribution
Flaviviridae	Yellow fever	Yellow fever virus	Mosquitoes	Africa, Caribbean, South America
	Dengue	Dengue virus serotypes 1–4	Mosquitoes	Americas, Asia, Oceania
Arenaviridae	Lassa fever	Lassa fever virus	None	West Africa
	Argentine haemorrhagic fever	Junin virus	None	Argentina
	Bolivian haemorrhagic fever	Machupo virus	None	Bolivia
	Venezuelan haemorrhagic fever	Guanarito virus	None	Venezuela
	Brazilian haemorrhagic fever	Sabia virus	None	Brazil
Bunyaviridae	Rift Valley fever	Rift Valley fever virus	Mosquitoes	East Africa, Arabian Peninsula
	Congo-Crimean haemorrhagic fever	Congo-Crimean haemorrhagic fever virus	Ticks	East Africa, Eastern Europe, Asia
	Haemorrhagic fever with renal syndrome	Hantaan, Seoul Dobrava viruses	None	Asia
	Nephropathia endemica	Puumala virus	None	Eastern Europe, Scandinavia, former Soviet Union
	Hantavirus pulmonary syndrome	Sin Nombre and Andes viruses	None	North and South America
Filoviridae	Marburg disease	Marburg	None	Africa
	Ebola haemorrhagic fever	Ebola virus (Zaire, Sudan and Côte d'Ivoire variants)	None	Africa

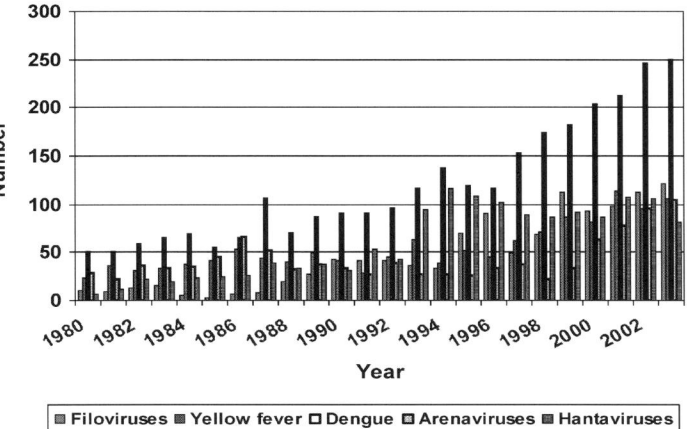

Fig. 1 Publications on selected viral haemorrhagic fevers recorded in the PubMed database of the National Library of Medicine, National Institutes of Health. Only citations in English have been recorded.

The causative agents of viral haemorrhagic fevers are distributed across four widely different RNA virus families (Table 1). These agents differ markedly in size, morphology, method of replication and interactions with the host. Yet all are capable of causing severe human disease manifested by a catastrophic failure of the vascular network and haematopoiesis. Interestingly, only a few viruses within each of these four families have such a capacity. Thus, there are several conundrums—what property or properties unite these virologically diverse agents to cause these similar clinical manifestations? And why do closely related viruses within the same family do not share the same propensity to cause severe clinical illness, if indeed they cause human disease at all?

What surely must be of concern is the all too likely scenario that other viruses with equal capacity to cause a serious outbreak of human disease may be misdiagnosed and thus go unrecognised in the critical early stages of an epidemic. Rapid air travel means that virus from a single index case can be spread in a matter of hours across three continents. The matter of laboratory diagnosis and confirmation of exotic infections have not been taken seriously by those responsible for public health and control. Development of new tests for early detection of viral haemorrhagic fevers and other emerging diseases is unfashionable with those administering peer review research funding and the commercial sector is reluctant to invest in developing assays for what it sees as a very restricted market opportunity in an era of increasingly heavy product regulation.

The burden of disease

The extent and scale of the prevalence, morbidity and mortality associated with viral haemorrhagic fevers are not well understood. Even in the developed world such assessments are often incomplete, and even when available often conflict with the short-term aspirations of politicians lacking the vision to appreciate the benefits afforded in the longer term by the planning and support of public health programmes. The perception of the general public at large is that infectious diseases are preventable and something more akin to the social ills of times past rather than a menace that threats a technologically advanced modern society. This mentality drives political policy to the extent that surveillance becomes starved of resources and in turn basic epidemiological information is at best unreliable and at worst lacking. It is against this backdrop of more needing to be done in terms of quantifying both the social and economic impact of these diseases especially in those countries where healthcare resources are scarce. WHO estimates that countries such as many small and impoverished nations in West Africa spend less than $20 per person on all aspects of medical care, a pitifully small sum considering the need for extensive childhood immunisation programmes and ignores the constant drain on resources presented by persisting disease. A case in point is Lassa fever, once thought to be a comparatively rare disease. Now recognised as surprisingly common in West Africa, McCormick et al. (1987a) have shown that Lassa fever is responsible for over 40% of all febrile adult admissions to hospitals in Sierra Leone and Liberia, and the most important cause of (medical) deaths in as many as 30%.

In the wider context of infectious disease research, infections that give rise to high morbidity and significant mortality in the developed world are priority candidates for public resources—the HIV epidemic is a clear example. In contrast, infections that are both rare and produce only mild illness and low mortality among the populations of the world's richest countries fall at the opposite end of the spectrum as far as funding agencies are concerned. The direct costs of treatment and control, together with the indirect costs associated with morbidity and loss of productive life, are quantifiable with an output that can be directly compared between diseases, both infectious and non-infectious. There have been moves to re-assess the likely economic impact and presumed economic benefits to be gained as a result of preventing infectious diseases, most notably by the United States' Institute of Medicine (Committee to Study Priorities for Vaccine Development, 2000). These studies show just how difficult it is to make the economic argument in support of disease prevention in developing countries where reliable estimates of direct and indirect costs are that much more difficult to obtain.

There is often a conflict between the priorities of international organisations such as the World Health Organisation and national needs. Globally, attention is often drawn to diseases that can spread easily, particularly by arthropods. Dengue fever is the prime example, representing as it does the most widespread of the viral haemorrhagic fevers, present on all major continents and affecting or threatening over 50 countries. In contrast, national and local health authorities may be more concerned with diseases of local importance, particularly zoonoses that are restricted to an animal reservoir limited in its distribution. Junin virus, the causative agent of AHF, is such an agent, being of considerable public health importance in Argentina but largely irrelevant elsewhere.

To an epidemiologist, it is the incidence of disease that determines its impact on a population, a parameter notoriously difficult to measure. Effective measurement of incidence requires good techniques for measuring antibody and virus detection, an infrastructure to ensure surveillance, and above all knowledgeable clinicians capable of differentiating viral haemorrhagic fevers from other febrile illnesses. Considerable data exists for disease caused by dengue and hantaviruses in the more economically developed regions, but as with all measurements of disease incidence, the only certainty is that there is extensive under-reporting. The question is: by how much? The official annual incidence of yellow fever in Central and South America is less than 1000 cases per year, but this number almost exclusively represents those fatal cases identified and detected by viscerotomy. Given a case fatality rate of 20%, the actual number of clinical cases is most likely to be far greater, most probably nearer 20 times the reported incidence (Monath, 2001). Data collected from Africa suggests that the degree of under-reporting is substantial, with up to 250 cases occurring for each officially reported case. For these reasons there has, until recently, been a mistaken perception that yellow fever is a comparatively rare disease. There is now an awakening realisation of yellow fever as a significant cause of morbidity, especially in Africa and South America. Only in the last decade has yellow fever vaccine been incorporated into childhood immunisation programmes in any meaningful way.

The economic impact of disease burden is almost impossible to assess in many regions where viral haemorrhagic fevers occur, particularly in terms of wage loss and a reduction in productivity. The duration of any temporary disability and the impact of social norms regarding the care of sick relatives are also difficult to quantify in fiscal terms, but are likely to be significant among the poorer nations. In terms of impact, the haemorrhagic fevers are intermediate between the flavivirus encephalitides, such as Japanese encephalitis, and self-limiting febrile illness. Monath (1985) some years ago attempted to estimate the socio-economic burden of yellow fever in West Africa, using a comparative analysis of "days of healthy life" previously applied in Ghana. This West African country suffers yellow fever outbreaks at regular intervals. One such epidemic occurred between 1977 and 1980, characterised by an attack rate of 20 per 100,000 of population. Monath estimated the total burden to be roughly that of cholera, venereal diseases or trypanosomiasis. If the undoubtedly high level of under-reporting were taken into account, yellow fever would rank as one of the most important cause of disease in West Africa. Although this analysis is somewhat dated, it shows that the socio-economic cost of yellow fever in the developing world is considerable. These conclusions can easily be applied to other infections, for example dengue, the most widespread of all the viral haemorrhagic fevers. Indeed, Monath makes the point that the case fatality ratio of dengue approaches cholera and polio. Lassa fever is a further example as to the difficulties in estimating the total burden of infection. McCormick et al. (1987b) found a surprisingly high proportion of febrile admissions to hospitals in Sierra Leone associated with Lassa fever. In this setting, the cost of keeping a patient in hospital for a week exceeds four times the average salary.

Despite the overwhelming case for investing adequately in public health infrastructure, there is an extreme reluctance on the part of governments to recognise the long-term value of such investment. The problem is exacerbated by incomplete data resulting from poor surveillance, adding fuel to the politician's argument that investment is not warranted owing to a lack of evidence. Political indifference in turn leads to a further decline in the very infrastructure needed to monitor infectious disease.

The changing environment

The environment in which we live is changing on an unprecedented scale. Approximately 25% of the Earth's rain forest has been cleared in the last 50 years, and greenhouse gases such as CO_2 have increased by 20% over the last two centuries. The net result of the greenhouse effect is to increase the surface temperature by around half a degree Celsius. This apparently trivial increase is an indicator of profound climatic change: global warming is linked with the melting of the polar caps and a continuous shift in weather patterns leading to sustained droughts and floods. Global warming is reshaping the environment and habitats of humans and wildlife. Mosquito vectors and rodent reservoirs are affected as a direct result of such swings in climatic conditions. Outbreaks of viral haemorrhagic fevers have been unequivocally associated with abnormal periods of drought, leading to unusually rapid increases in rodent numbers. This upsurge in turn increases considerably the risk of human exposure to the pathogens they carry and furthers the opportunity that viral genomes vary as the ecology of their hosts changes. This can lead to altered patterns of disease. To some extent, the emergence of viral diseases—particularly the viral haemorrhagic fevers—are warning signs that serious perturbations of our ecosystems are happening. It is sobering that there has been at least one new disease coming to our attention every year for the last decade (Table 2).

The relentless change inflicted by humans on habitats in the name of progress has had a marked effect on rodent habitats. Over the last 50 years, nearly a quarter of the world's forests have disappeared to make way for intensive agriculture, mining, roads and other artefacts of human existence. Murine species are more resistant and adaptable than most. Whilst other rodent genera have declined, murine rodents have expanded in population size, especially in peri-urban areas. This resilience is immediately evident by casual observation from the platforms of any subway system in a major capital city. What this means is that, although species diversity has become less with fewer genera represented, those remaining have thrived; in most instances these are murine rodents, the species most likely to harbour zoonoses.

Table 2

Newly emerging viruses since 1990: viruses given in italics are considered as viral haemorrhagic fevers

Year	Virus	Country	Features
1990	*Guanarito virus*	Venezuela	Haemorrhagic disease, first thought to be dengue
1993	*Sin Nombre virus*	USA	Hantavirus Pulmonary Ssyndrome (HPS)
1994	*Sabia virus*	Brazil	Laboratory infection
	Alkhurma virus	Saudi Arabia	Outbreak in butchers
1995	Hendra virus	Australia	New paramyxovirus discovered in flying foxes
	Whitewater Arroyo virus	USA	Severe human disease
1996	*Andes virus*	Argentina	New pathogenic hantavirus
1997	Nipah virus	Malaysian peninsula	New paramyxovirus discovered in pigs
2002	SARS coronavirus	China, SE Asia	Acute respiratory disease

Of all the member species of the mammalian order Rodentia, it is members of the family Muridae that has been most successful and are to be found in almost all habitats. This family has species that are the natural hosts of almost all arenaviruses and hantaviruses. Importantly, these species are susceptible to climate and ecological change, resulting in variable population numbers. Rodents belonging to the family Muridae appear to have undergone most of their evolutionary history in the Old World, arriving in the New World comparatively recently via the Bering land isthmus some 20–30 million years ago. It is these more recent arrivals into South America that represent the reservoirs of arenaviruses and hantaviruses.

The influence of climate changes on wild rodent populations can be considerable. Fluctuations in population sizes occur in regular cycles, particularly in arid and semi-arid zones where small climate changes can bring about significant fluctuations in food quality and quantity. The extent of such variations is magnified when there are abnormal weather patterns. The most potent climatic driver of environmental change is the so-called "El Niño—Southern Oscillation (ENSO)" centred on an irregular pattern of atmospheric and oceanic current conditions along the Pacific seaboard of South America. These trigger aberrant weather patterns ranging from extreme arid periods to abnormal rainfall, the latter resulting in floods and explosive increases in arthropod and rodent populations. The sudden expansion in number of deer mice that immediately preceded the 1993 Four Corners emergence of HPS has been blamed on abnormal rainfall resulting from changes in the El Nino system. Thus, the risk of vector borne disease and zoonoses are exacerbated, often in areas where the medical infrastructure is fragile even in times of stability. The emergence of Machupo virus (Bolivian haemorrhagic fever) in the Beni region of North East Bolivia in the 1960s was linked to a sudden rise in the numbers of *Calomys callosus* that followed an abnormally dry period, this exacerbated by a drop in the number of feral cats as a result of the widespread use of DDT.

Those diseases requiring an arthropod vector for transmission between reservoir and humans can emerge suddenly after heavy rainfall, especially if transovarial transmission maintains the virus in the environment during dry periods. The relationship between a virus and its arthropod vector is more than just regarding the insect acting as a mechanical vehicle for transferring virus from one host to another. A well-established biological relationship evolves in a way that the vector plays a major role in the evolution of the virus and adaptation of the virus to a changing ecology. Present thinking is that viruses evolve to the point where there is a steady-state relationship between virus and vector, and virus and host. Any perturbation in the vector, host or genome thus would imbalance these equilibria, leading to the emergence or re-emergence of disease.

The importance of surveillance

The monitoring of infectious disease outbreaks normally rests with national authorities charged with assessing individual cases for cause, and compiling population-based epidemiological data. The move to centralise diagnostic facilities mitigates against sustaining a competence in recognising those unusual clinical cases that may herald an outbreak of something new and more dangerous than the normal run of febrile illness.

All experts in the control of infectious diseases agree that effective control requires the engagement of multidisciplinary teams spearheaded by alert clinicians. Experience from many outbreaks shows clearly the need for veterinarians, epidemiologists and ecologists to work in concert with microbiologists. This has been amply shown by the experience of agencies in the USA in controlling the West Nile incursion into North America in 1999. Failure to integrate these disciplines can have disastrous consequences.

The four cornerstones for controlling viral haemorrhagic fevers, and indeed any emerging disease, are:

1. *Alert clinicians with easy access to local laboratories and pathology services*: Training in infectious disease control has suffered in many regions over the last two decades, with continuing professional development often neglecting the more traditional approach of sharpening clinical skills backed by a sound knowledge of pathogen diagnosis, pathology and epidemiology. Rationalisation of laboratories in developed countries has continued unabated, with the result that all too often microbiologists at a local level are poorly equipped to recognise the first signs of disease outbreaks and react accordingly.

2. *Good serology provided by national reference laboratories*: Keeping stocks of characterised and standardised reagents is crucial. Almost all of the viral haemorrhagic fever outbreaks recorded in recent years have been diagnosed rapidly and accurately by antibody detection assays for which remain the most relevant of all the presently available methods. Although genome-specific assays employing PCR technology are increasingly used as soon as is practicable, such assays are fraught with difficulties relating to specificity and sensitivity. Sample collection is frequently not performed with the degree of rigour necessary to avoid the confusion that can result from sample contamination.

3. *Involvement of epidemiologists and communicable disease specialists at the earliest possible opportunity*: Increasingly sophisticated mathematical modelling of disease outbreaks brings insight into the transmissibility kinetics and offers time-saving pointers to effective containment and control. In the case of vector borne disease, the use of satellite images to detect climate-induced changes in vegetation patterns also enhances the accuracy of these models. If vaccines are available, the application of sound epidemiological principles is essential in order that an adequate level of herd immunity is attained as quickly as possible.

4. *The ability to deliver effective and prompt control measures*: Time and time again outbreaks of severe diseases such as Ebola and Lassa fever have been inflamed by inadequate control procedures and, when implemented, often too late in the day for effective containment. The outbreak of Ebola in the Sudan in 1996 was controlled largely by closing the hospitals at the centre of the outbreak combined with the meticulous tracking and isolation of contacts and family members. Recent experience with SARS has shown vividly how nosocomial outbreaks of disease may occur even in the best equipped and staffed hospital settings.

To the above could be added the necessity of engaging veterinarians, especially where zoonotic disease is suspected. The 1999 West Nile outbreak in the USA showed how valuable time can be lost when the first signs of disease incursion are seen in wild and domestic animals. Traditionally, there has been little effort to integrate human and veterinary public health, yet the principles and practice of disease control are broadly the same regardless of the target species. New pathogens have come to light almost annually since the early 1990s, many associated with domesticated species and livestock.

Although outside the brief of most microbiologists, the handling of the press and other media can take a heavy toll on those directly involved in controlling an outbreak. Specialists in media relations can be of considerable help, not only in controlling news flow but also in communicating to the public at large the degree of risk individual circumstances may present, and the tracing of potential contacts. News media are often badly informed as is graphically illustrated by the continued use by British tabloid journalists of the term Green Monkey Disease for filovirus infections; despite the fact that such monkeys are not known to be susceptible to either Ebola or Marburg viruses. Yet a fully informed and briefed press can play an important role in containing the spread of disease in the community. As with many aspects of science, there is a reluctance of microbiologists and medical personnel alike to engage the media. Experts in infectious disease control frequently lack the skills and motivation to ensure journalists understand the issues of the moment. Failure to do so invites the misinterpretation of events and ignores a vital channel of communicating essential information to the public at large. Media training as an essential element of infectious disease education is long overdue.

The use of the web has transformed communications between professionals and the public alike. Used responsibly, secure websites dedicated to the recording and dissemination of data can do much to alert clinicians, microbiologists and public health officials with responsibility for containing an outbreak. Health care professionals in the developing world frequently are in a position that, for them, access to the Internet is easier than obtaining printed journals and reports. To this end, the World Health Organisation, the Food and Agricultural Organisation, and Centers for Disease Control maintain excellent portals for accessing disease control protocols and information.

A further issue is the preparedness of government agencies to maintain isolation facilities and disease control capability in prolonged periods between outbreaks. Governments become lulled into a sense of false security and come reluctant to sustain expensive facilities. An example was the decision of the Victorian State Government in Australia to close the isolation facilities at the Fairfield Hospital in Melbourne, despite vigorous advice to the contrary from infectious disease experts worldwide. Just a few years later, new morbilliviruses were isolated in Queensland that could have easily presented a new public health threat to much of Australia. Governments are traditionally myopic as to the true costs of disease. For example, WHO estimates that the actual cost of the BSE crisis in the UK to exceed around $32 billion.

Viral haemorrhagic fevers at a glance

All of the viral haemorrhagic fevers possess certain common features (Table 3). With the exception of hantavirus infections, clinical disease correlates with the period of virus circulation in the blood. This has implications both for diagnosis and for the handling of samples as well as for the isolation of infected individuals. All begin with an insidious acute febrile phase. Patients present with myalgia and malaise, progressing to prostration. The challenge for the attending physician is distinguishing the early stages of viral haemorrhagic fevers from the onset of other, invariably more common, causes of febrile illness such as influenza and malaria. Individuals themselves may delay seeking medical attention thus increasing the risk of spread to family and close contacts, as occurred during the outbreak of Ebola haemorrhagic fever in the Sudan in 1977. It is only towards the end of the 3–4 day acute phase that signs of any vascular disturbance become apparent.

Vascular permeability due to damage of the vascular endothelium is accompanied by a precipitate drop in platelet count and often a marked reduction in leucocytes. A thrombocytopenia is particularly indicative of viral haemorrhagic fever. The disease process is poorly understood although we are now beginning to understand more concerning the interactions between viral proteins and the cells they infect. Vascular endothelium is particularly susceptible to a surge in chemokine and cytokine levels triggered by virus replication. Most viral haemorrhagic fevers are directly cytolytic for the cells they infect, leading to rapid loss of organ function. The exceptions are the hantaviruses and dengue where the immune response plays a major role in the pathological process. In general, viral haemorrhagic fevers are multi-organ diseases and pantropic in their effects.

It is critical that a presumptive diagnosis is arrived at as early as possible. Thus, a complete patient history is essential to aid the differential diagnosis from other causes of febrile illness (Table 4). An accurate travel history recording countries visited and whether the patient has visited rural areas. Vaccination status for yellow fever needs to be checked in the traveller who has returned from South or Central America, or West Africa.

Table 3

Similarities and differences among the viral haemorrhagic fevers

	Similarities	Differences
Virology	Enveloped viruses	Virion structure
	Small single stranded RNA genomes	Distinct mechanisms of gene expression and replication
		Inhibition by ribavirin
Epidemiology	Aerosol infectivity	Vectors and animal hosts
	Persist in the environment	Geographical distribution
Pathology	Causes vascular dysfunction	Pathogenesis
	Sensitivity to interferon	Host immune responses
		Cytopathic effects on mammalian cells

Table 4

Factors to be considered in the early stages of diagnosis

Clinical history: factors to be considered
Travel to tropical/endemic areas? If so, time of arrival and departure
Has the patient visited sick relatives, family or friends whilst away?
Did the visit include excursions into rural areas?
Has there been a known exposure to ticks, wild animals or rodents?
Has the patient been vaccinated against yellow fever?

Detailed information on current outbreaks can be found on many national and international websites (see Appendix 1 for further details). Travellers restricting their visits to major cities are unlikely to encounter the pathogens described in this book, most of which are essentially confined to rural areas. The exception is those who visit family and friends in hospitals within endemic areas: as many viral haemorrhagic fever outbreaks have been associated with inadequate isolation of infected patients, the true nature of the infection having escaped recognition on admission.

Patients with a history of contact with wild animals and peridomestic rodents are particularly at risk. Those with evidence of tick bite could have been exposed to agents such as Congo-Crimean haemorrhagic fever or Omsk haemorrhagic fever. Unfortunately exposure to mosquitoes is so common to make the patient recounting of mosquito bites unhelpful, although the season of travel is relevant as many of the viral haemorrhagic fevers cause epidemics during or immediately after heavy rainfall.

The recording of arrival and departure dates is important to establish the likelihood of a patient being within the incubation period of a particular infection. Patients presenting more than 3 weeks after returning from an endemic area are most unlikely to have contracted a viral haemorrhagic fever and other causes should be suspected. Even an individual having visited a rural area and presenting with an acute febrile illness within a few days of return may not necessarily be incubating a viral haemorrhagic fever if they have spent some time within a major city before their return flight. Many patients have not received prompt attention for malaria owing to delays in preparing and examining a blood smear.

The rapid adoption of rigorous barrier nursing procedures coupled with the handling of clinical specimens under containment conditions can do much to alleviate the heightened risks that are present before a definitive diagnosis is made. Viral haemorrhagic fevers are extremely dangerous and, wherever there is doubt, immediate advice should be sought from national and international authorities.

Scope of the book

Each of the following chapters contains self-contained descriptions of the major causes of viral haemorrhagic fevers, grouped according to families. The properties of each virus are outlined in relation to epidemiology, clinical presentation and treatment. Each is preceded by an overview of the molecular properties and replication. This is a rapidly expanding area, however, thus the virology of each infection is presented more in a manner intended to provide the reader with an overview prior to delving more fully into the original references. Where appropriate, a brief historical backdrop can be found as many early pioneers in this field have done much to inform and shape our present thinking as to how best these infections can be controlled and treated.

The final chapter attempts to place the viral haemorrhagic fevers in the broader context of infectious disease control and prevention. In particular, the potential threat from the use of these viruses as agents of terror is commented upon with some suggestions as to how best this threat may be countered. The emphasis throughout is to develop an understanding as to the nature of this rather disparate collection of human pathogens, through an integrated approach of clinical diagnosis, pathology, epidemiology and virology.

The number of references has been kept to a minimum in order to ease the reader through the chapters as ready access to web-based literature databases now permits more exhaustive literature reviews than can possibly be presented in a single monograph. A guide to obtaining further information on the worldwide web is given in Appendix 1. Appendix 2 summarises various sources of further reading, including more populist works that have been written for the general public, many of which contain useful sources of information for the specialist and thus should not be ignored. Finally Appendix 3 offers a brief description as to the different containment levels as applied to laboratories and associated facilities.

Flaviviruses

The family Flaviridae contains more than 70 members, many responsible for a considerable proportion of mortality and mortality worldwide, both in humans and animals. The family is divided into three genera: flavivirus, pestivirus and hepacivirus. The biological properties of each genus are distinct, although all share similar structural characteristics and genome organisation. Members of the genus flavivirus have a worldwide distribution although individual viruses are invariably restricted by climate and vector. More than half of the genus flavivirus are associated with human disease, including yellow fever virus, the prototype virus of the genus and an important cause of viral haemorrhagic fever. Other important pathogens in the genus include Japanese encephalitis virus found in Southeast Asia and tick-borne encephalitis virus present in Europe and Northern Asia.

The majority of the viruses in the genus flavivirus are arboviruses—transmitted between mammalian hosts by an invertebrate vector (mosquitoes and ticks). Virus replication takes place in both the vertebrate host and the insect vector. In the case of yellow fever and dengue viruses, these are maintained in the wild by transmission from primates to mosquitoes, and back to primates. Humans are infected as accidental event when intruding into this natural ecosystem. Dengue virus has evolved along with the expansion of major conurbations to the extent that some experts argue a sylvatic cycle through an animal reservoir is no longer necessary for its endemicity.

Flavivirus distribution is dependent on the ecology of their vertebrate and invertebrate hosts. Thus, some have a very restricted geographical distribution, e.g. Omsk haemorrhagic fever is restricted to western Siberia and Kyasanur Forest disease is found so far only in Karnataka (Mysore) state of India. The recent emergence of Alkhurma virus on the Arabian Peninsula is a puzzle, as this virus clearly shows a relationship with Kyasanur Forest virus. Dengue has expanded over the last 20 years from southeast Asia into the Pacific, the Americas, Africa and Australia, progressively establishing itself in local populations of the ubiquitous *Aedes aegypti*. The rapid expansion of dengue virus coupled to the increasing incidence of dengue shock syndrome and haemorrhagic fever makes this infection a global priority in terms of control and public health. Dengue is regarded as one of the top priorities for public resources by the tropical disease programme of the World Health Organisation.

The ecology of *A. aegypti* plays a critical part in the epidemiology of both yellow fever and dengue. *A. aegypti* is unusually small compared to other mosquitoes and is well adapted to virus transmission. It rarely circulates beyond human habitation and is unusually silent in flight, meaning that the female can often seek a blood meal unnoticed, aiming particularly for uncovered legs and ankles. The female can survive for many months, sometimes for a year or even longer. Transovarial passage of the virus from adult to egg ensures that the virus can survive throughout a dry season. Flaviviruses replicate in the salivary glands and are introduced into a new human host together with saliva. Again in contrast to other mosquitoes, *A. aegypti* lays its eggs individually, dispersed over large areas of still water: this maximises the chance of survival. Although the female avoids dirty or polluted water, eggs can survive in water that has been chlorinated.

Outbreaks of flavivirus infections often coincide with climatic events, for example, heavy rain following a period of drought. This results in numerous stagnant pools, ideal breeding grounds for both mosquitoes and ticks.

Surveillance and epidemiological monitoring are essential for the prevention and management of flavivirus infections. Continual and sustained sampling of arthropod vectors and vertebrate hosts for arbovirus activity is required to ensure such surveillance remains effective. Unfortunately, there has been all too often a heavy reliance on initiating mosquito eradication programmes without due regard for subsequent monitoring of disease and vector absence. The result is that some countries within endemic areas have all but ceased to monitor for outbreaks. Active surveillance can also provide early indications as to the emergence of arboviral and other diseases: Venezuela had ceased surveillance for some years but the emergence of Venezuelan haemorrhagic fever in the 1980s illustrated vividly the need for continual surveillance. This hitherto unrecognised disease was first attributed to dengue virus but more detailed epidemiological investigation uncovered the presence of Guanarito virus, a member of the Arenaviridae family (see Arenaviruses).

Clinical manifestations of the majority of flavivirus infections are relatively non-specific. In endemic areas, diagnosis is often based on clinical suspicion, especially if the attending physician is alerted by epidemic activity in the region. Scarce or non-existent resources in economically underdeveloped regions compound the difficulties in obtaining accurate and detailed data. For some years, the Rockefeller Foundation sponsored the surveillance for yellow fever in South America by providing equipment for collecting liver samples from deceased individuals suspected of having had yellow fever. Fixed tissue sections were then transported to regional laboratories for further analyses. This initiative was the exception, however, and sustained monitoring of yellow fever and other indigenous diseases remains as problematical as ever.

Yellow fever is the only viral haemorrhagic disease against which a vaccine is widely available for human use. Indeed, the 17D yellow fever vaccine has been extraordinarily successful. In contrast, the development of vaccines against dengue virus has been fraught with difficulties, despite the many similarities of these two viruses. The success and failures of developing flavivirus vaccines serve as useful paradigms for the development of rational vaccines against viral haemorrhagic fevers and other exotic infections.

There are many excellent reviews of flaviviruses. Particularly useful as to the scope of the problems these viruses present are the overviews on yellow fever by Monath (2001) and on dengue by Gubler (2002). The World Health Organisation and the United States Centres for Disease control maintain useful websites on dengue (http://www.who.int/health-topics/dengue and http://www.cdc.gov/ncidod/dvbid/dengue).

Yellow fever

Historical background

Yellow fever is regarded as one of the classic diseases of antiquity, instilling dread and terror in the Americas, Europe and Africa in the three centuries following the arrival of the Spanish conquistadors in the New World. The cause remained a mystery until the work of Walter Reed and his team in Cuba in 1900 proved transmission by *A. aegypti*.

Through the 18th and 19th centuries the colonisation of the Americas was retarded by frequent outbreaks of yellow fever. The Philadelphia outbreak of 1793 was one of many epidemics that hit the then capital of the United States in its infancy. The outbreak was particularly severe, affecting over 10% of the city's 40,000 population. The source was most likely arriving on boats from the West Indies fleeing the yellow fever outbreak of the preceding year. Rudimentary efforts at quarantine[1] failed to stop the epidemic, which was widely believed to be linked to rotting coffee, waste or putrid air.

The outbreak could not have come at a worse time for the fledgling United States. Philadelphia was at this time the seat of government but the city had to be all but abandoned by George Washington and his administration. The epidemic began in August: by October of 1793 over 5000 out of a total population of 55,000 had succumbed, with 6000 inhabitants ill at any one time. In the midst of this epidemic, Benjamin Rush (Fig. 1) promoted a savage regimen of bleeding and purging, accompanied by massive doses of calomel. Rush, who we will meet later in the section on dengue, was both a prominent physician and one of the signatories to the Declaration of Independence. Rush subscribed heavily to the miasma theory of disease, pinpointing a spoiled load of coffee left on the city's wharves as the likely source of the outbreak. The views held by Rush eventually became entwined with his republicanism, and his counsel as to how best patients should be treated acquired increasingly partisan overtones. The political paralysis resulting from the 1793 outbreak is believed by historians to have contributed significantly to the neutralist stance of the newly emerging nation at a time when there was intense political manoeuvring to have the United States declare support for France in its war against England. Indeed, recurring epidemics of yellow fever did much over the ensuing century to shape the United States, especially given the disruptive effect of the disease on commerce and settlement of the southern states.

Yellow fever is the archetypal haemorrhagic fever. It brought fear into the hearts of the early African explorers and its carriage across the Atlantic as a consequence of the slave trade did much to shape the European settlement of the New World. It emerged first in the ports of West Africa, then on slave trading vessels, to arrive finally in the Caribbean. This process took nearly a century after the Americas were first discovered, most likely because of the length of the sea voyage. An acute infection is dependent upon mosquitoes for transmission, and those persons infected before departure succumbed well before landfall. Only by maintaining the transmission cycle several times via shipboard

[1] The term quarantine is derived from the Italian *quaranta*, meaning 40 days, a measure first introduced by the Venetian Republic in 1374.

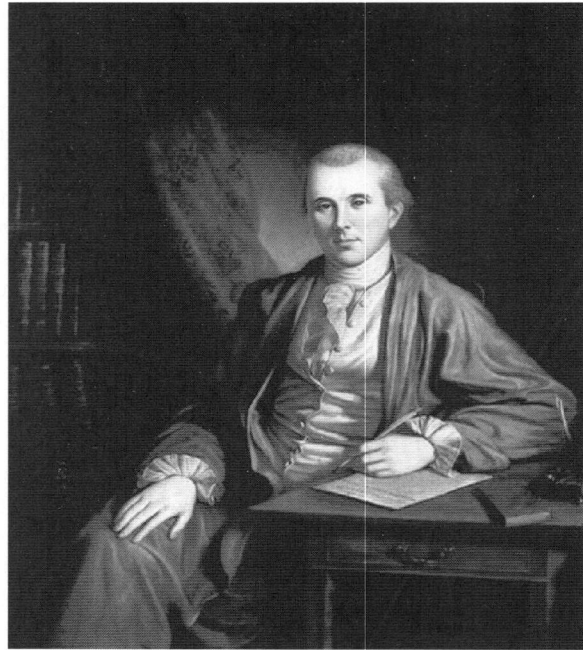

Fig. 1 Benjamin Rush (1745–1813), American Founding Father and Physician.

mosquitoes could the virus survive the 10–12 week crossing, and only then if the crew and passengers survived. There is a contrary view that yellow fever moved from the Americas to Africa based on accounts of a disease resembling yellow fever before Europeans reached the New World. This is highly unlikely, especially given the high susceptibility of the indigenous population of the time and the susceptibility of New World monkeys to yellow fever virus. This susceptibility of New World primates to yellow fever virus contrasts sharply with the situation among Old World monkeys where yellow fever virus is very much in equilibrium with its animal reservoirs. There is a myth that Africans are less susceptible to yellow fever virus, but the reality is that yellow fever is part of the normal repertoire of infectious diseases that children are exposed to and from which recovery is the normal outcome. Thus, much of the indigenous population acquires immunity in the first years of life that extends into adulthood.

Yellow fever first appeared in 1647 in Barbados, quickly spreading to other parts of the Caribbean and the Yucatan Peninsula. Over the next two centuries it spread throughout Central America, south to Brazil and as far north as New York and Boston. European ports also suffered when ships berthed on return from the Americas. The effect on troops and settlers in the Caribbean was particularly devastating. In 1655 France sent a force of around 1500 men to take St Lucia from the British but only 89 survived the ravages of yellow fever and other diseases. Nearly a century later, the English Admiral Vernon in 1741 lost nearly half of a 19,000 strong force intent on taking Cartegena in present-day Columbia perished as a direct result of the disease.

In the closing years of the 19th century the United States government decided it was high time to root out the cause of yellow fever. The germ theory of disease had begun to be widely accepted and new causes of infectious disease were being described with almost monotonous regularity. The Surgeon General thus dispatched Walter Reed in 1899 to newly conquered Cuba. There he was joined among others by Carlos Finlay. Carlos Finlay, born of Scots and French parents, had experienced at first-hand the tragic effects of yellow fever when training in Philadelphia in 1853.

Reed and his colleagues first explored a bacterium proposed earlier by Giuseppe Sanarelli as the likely agent: this soon proved a false trail, however, with this bacterium subsequently being linked to hog cholera. Given the ascendancy and zeal of bacteriologists at the time, Reed and his fellow investigators were under considerable pressure to confirm a bacterium as the cause. How Reed and his team hit upon the concept of insect transmission is one of the great debates of medical endeavour. The widely quoted view is that Reed was aware of the work emanating from Ronald Ross in China whose studies on malarial transmission by mosquitoes were published a few years earlier in 1897. Two British physicians working in Havana at the same time as Reed almost certainly drew Reed's attention to the study of Ross. Reed made the connection, perhaps, that yellow fever often occurred when malaria was also prevalent. But the input of Carlos Finlay also needs acknowledging as he was aware of the investigations of Patrick Manson who described the role of mosquitoes in transmitting filariasis years earlier. Indeed mosquito transmission had been suggested as early as 1807 by John Crawford of Baltimore, a hypothesis reiterated by Joshua Nott in 1848. However the concept originated, Reed and his co-workers set up carefully controlled experiments, the outcome of which demonstrated unambiguously the role of mosquitoes in the transmission of yellow fever. Importantly for the time, they also showed that the agent was a "filterable virus" and not a bacterium.

Reed's work in Cuba led to intensive efforts to controlling urban yellow fever by reducing opportunities for individuals to be bitten by infected *Aedes* mosquitoes. Notwithstanding rural infections continued to occur and in response the Rockefeller Foundation's Commission for International Health embarked upon a programme of global eradication. To this end, the Commission went to Guayacil in Ecuador where yellow fever was still very much in evidence. Hideyo Noguchi soon reported he had isolated the causative organism in guinea pigs, calling it *Leptospira icteroides*. He raised a therapeutic antiserum which he persuaded himself and those around him to have the properties of a passive prophylactic.

Doubts as to the cause of yellow fever lingered, however, and in the early 1920s the Commission decided to re-evaluate the cause of yellow fever, but this time focusing efforts on West Africa, long regarded as the source of the disease. A permanent research station was established at Yaba, close to Lagos, and it was there that Adrian Stokes, an Irish physician appointed in 1922 to the chair in pathology at Guy's Hospital Medical School, successfully showed the viral nature of yellow fever by transmission to crown monkeys (*Macacus simicus*) from India using field isolates from Latch near Accra in present-day Ghana. After an incubation period of 2–6 days a period of high fever followed leading to eventually to collapse and death. Pathological changes were reproducible and re-transmission occurred after passing monkey serum from acutely ill animals through Berkefield filters. This early work in Ghana has recently been reviewed by Mortimer (2002).

This important work established the foundations whereby Sawyer in New York was able to develop what we now know as the 17D vaccine strains of yellow fever virus. Tragically Adrian Stokes succumbed to yellow fever, as had Noguchi, in Accra in 1928. These strategies prompted transferral of further work to the comparatively more controlled environment of New York.

Yellow fever continued to frustrate the aspirations of Europeans in settling and exploiting the Americas and Africa until well into the 20th century. It was common for seaman to become infected visiting the shorelines of these tropical zones but the victims inevitably perished at sea. The mosquitoes were hardier, however, and transovarial transmission ensured that infected insects could come ashore once ships had berthed in the northern hemisphere. One such episode occurred in September 1865 when the barque "Hecla" docked in Swansea when the weather was unseasonably warm (Meers, 1986). The "Hecla" had loaded a cargo of copper ore in Cuba as well as infected mosquitoes. Despite deaths amongst the crew whilst en route, the captain did not quarantine the ship before berthing. The result was a total of 27 infections and 15 deaths amongst those of the local population living or working within 200 m of the "Hecla". Detailed weather records are available, and show that a dip in day time temperatures below 17–18°C for 3 days arrested the epidemic. Meers estimates that a maximum of 10 infected mosquitoes would have sufficed to cause this local outbreak. Although the diagnosis at this time would have been entirely on clinical observations, this outbreak almost certainly was due to yellow fever. It illustrates vividly how readily arboviruses can be transmitted across oceans, as was seen again as recently as 1999 when West Nile virus was introduced into the USA.

Epidemiology

Yellow fever is confined to the tropical regions of Africa and the Americas. Persistence of the disease is dependent upon cyclical transmission between monkeys and humans with mosquitoes as vectors. Thus, the epidemiology of the disease is driven by a series of complex interactions between the virus, its arthropod vectors and reservoir hosts.

These interactions give rise to two discrete transmission cycles, with marked variations between the cycles in Africa and South America. These interactions are summarised in Fig. 2.

Sylvatic, or "jungle" cycle

In forested areas, monkeys are the principal reservoirs, although infections in non-human primates tend to be transient and thus any viraemia is relatively short lived. The cycle

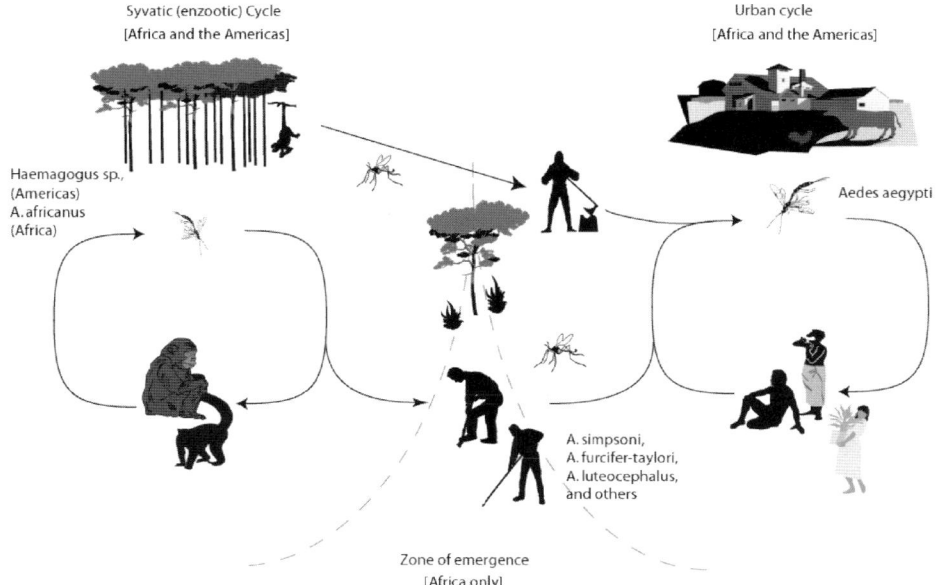

Fig. 2 Transmission cycles of yellow fever.

differs between the Old and New Worlds both in terms of the species of monkeys infected, the outcome of this infection in primates and the mosquito vectors involved in transmission.

In Africa, yellow fever virus infects principally *Cerepithecus* and *Colobus* species, and in West Africa is transmitted by either *Aedes furcifer-taylori* or *Aedes luteocephalus*. In East and Central Africa the cycle is maintained principally by *Aedes simpsoni*. African non-human primates are relatively resistant to the infection and most recover. The associated viraemia is relatively short lived and therefore the chances of mosquito transmission are lessened. The distinct nature of the cycle between West and East Africa reflects the evolution of yellow fever virus in association with its host over a long period of time. These profiles are in accord with the distinctive genotypes of yellow fever virus recovered from patients in these different localities on the African continent.

In South America the sylvatic cycle is quite distinct. The virus is found in *Aloutta*, *Ateles*, *Callethrix*, *Cebus* and *Saimiri* monkeys and is frequently lethal. Widespread outbreaks occur centred on the river basin draining the Amazonian rain forest. Current thinking is that the virus was introduced into the rain forest ecosystem from urban outbreaks, aided by the adaptation of yellow fever virus to several species of tree-dwelling *Haemagogus* mosquitoes. As in the African cycle, mosquitoes remain infected for life once having bitten an infected monkey, with the virus passing transovarially to larvae. Humans only become infected by the bites of such insects on clearing trees or if the insect population spills over at the margins of forested areas into rural communities.

Human infections once initiated can instigate human-to-human transmission independent of the monkey population in the immediate environment. This is increasingly the case in Africa where the monkey populations have declined as human modification of their habitat has accelerated.

The margins of forest and savannah in Africa give rise to zones of emergence where during the rainy season the chance of human infection intensifies as vector numbers dramatically increase, only to decline once more during the dry season. It is at these margins, particularly after prolonged drought, that yellow fever re-emerges with serious consequences, especially among children with no immunity.

The urban cycle

This is maintained by peri-domestic mosquitoes such as *A. aegypti*. Efforts to eradicate this vector in Central and South America in the second half of the 20th century were largely successful in ensuring urban areas became free of yellow fever. Cessation of mosquito eradication programmes out of environmental concerns, however, has resulted in insect levels being restored to near pre-eradication levels in many areas. As yet, there has not been a resurgence of urban yellow fever in the Americas, mainly as a result of vigorous vaccination programmes. Humans entering forested areas infested by virus carrying infected mosquitoes become bitten by female insects. These live from 70 to 160 days and have a flight range of over 300 m. Eggs are laid in still water, and can be disseminated readily in pots, crevasses and old car tires.

In recent decades, yellow fever has been a far bigger public health problem in Africa, a continent where mosquito eradication has not been widely practiced and immunisation tends not to be widespread. The size and frequency of outbreaks in Africa varies between West Africa, and Central and East Africa. Outbreaks in East Africa are generally few and far between, although the largest outbreak ever recorded occurred in southwestern Ethiopia in 1960–1962, claiming around 30,000 lives with more than 100,000 people infected. This outbreak had a severe impact in such a sparsely populated region of less than one million. With the exception of the 1986–1988 outbreaks in Nigeria when over 44,000 cases were recorded, outbreaks in West Africa have occurred more often but tend to be limited in scope. Yellow fever has gradually spread from countries such as Côte D'Ivoire, Burkino Faso and Cameroon to Gabon, Liberia and Kenya, countries thought to be free of infection before the middle of the 20th century.

Properties of yellow fever virus

Morphology

Virions are spherical and approximately 50 nm in diameter with an outer lipid membrane enclosing an inner nucleocapsid (Fig. 3). Mature virions contain two membrane proteins, E and M. Detailed structure analysis of tick-borne encephalitis virus has revealed, for this flavivirus at least, that the E protein is arranged as dimers orientated

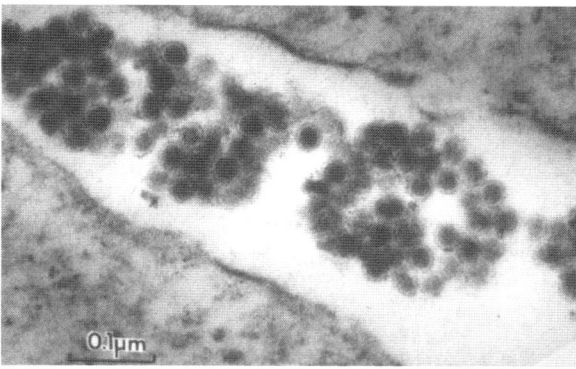

Fig. 3 Morphogenesis of yellow fever virus within infected Vero cells (Ishak et al., 1988).

parallel to the membrane surface. Thus, the flaviviruses do not show surface projections as is often the case for enveloped virus, such as influenza (family Myxoviridae) and rabies (family Rhabdoviridae). Both the arrangement of these dimers and the underlying nucleocapsid conform to the principles of icosahedral symmetry. Immature virions differ in that prM protein replaces the M protein.

Genetic organisation and gene expression

The flavivirus genome is an approximately 11 kb RNA molecule of positive sense[2] with respect to protein translation. The 5′ end of the genome possess a type I cap (m-7GpppAmp) followed by the conserved dinucleotide AG. Flavivirus genomes are the only positive stranded RNA viruses of mammals that do not possess a poly(A) tract at the 3′ end: the 3′ terminus ends with the conserved dinucleotide CU. While nucleotide sequences are divergent amongst members of the flavivirus genus, the secondary structures at the 5′ and 3′ ends are conserved among mosquito-borne and tick-borne members of the genus.

In common with the picornaviruses, the viral genes are first expressed by synthesis of a large polyprotein (Fig. 4). This single precursor molecule then undergoes a series of cleavages thereby generating functional proteins. Cleavages are mediated either by the host signal peptidase present in the lumen of the endoplasmic reticulum or by a viral serine protease. The 5′ and 3′ ends of the genome are not translated, the secondary structure in this region having a role in mediating genome replication.

---

[2] By convention, the nucleic acid strand coding directly for protein is referred to as the positive strand (i.e. is of positive polarity). The complementary sequence of nucleotide bases arising from the replication process cannot be used directly for protein synthesis and is thus of negative sense with respect to ribosomal translation (i.e. is of negative polarity).

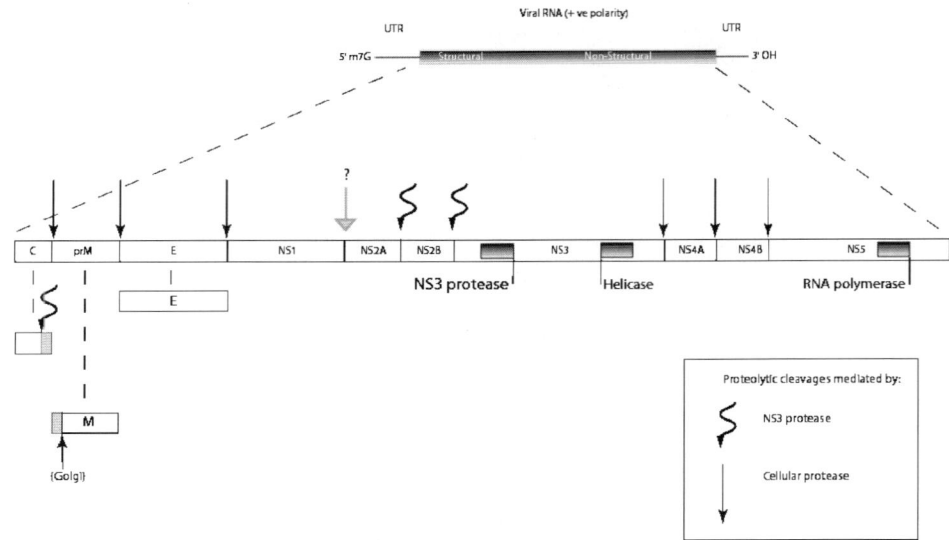

Fig. 4 Organisation of the yellow fever genome.

Gene expression starts by ribosomes binding to a site downstream from the 5′ terminus, bypassing several AUG initiation codons before recognising a site close to the AUG located immediately upstream of the capsid, C gene. This internal ribosome entry event required for translating the viral genome is common to both flaviviruses and picornaviruses: the internal ribosome binding entry site (IRES) is formed in part by the secondary structure of the 5′ non-translated region.

A total of 10 proteins are expressed as a result of the processing of the polyprotein precursor. The three structural proteins, capsid (C), membrane (prM/M) and envelope (E) are expressed at the 5′ end, followed by the genes coding for the non-structural proteins, NS1, NS2A, NS2B, NS3, NS4A, NS4B and NS5 (Fig. 4). Polyprotein processing confers the advantage that gene expression can be controlled by the rate and extent to which these cleavage events occur. In addition, the use of alternative cleavage sites results in proteins with stretches of amino acid homology but different functions. This form of viral protein synthesis is likely inefficient, however, with some gene products being produced surplus to the requirements of virus replication.

Structural proteins

The two viral envelope proteins, E and M, are type I integral membrane proteins with C-terminal anchor sequences. By analogy with tick-borne encephalitis virus, the E protein consists predominantly of β-sheets arranged in a head-to-tail configuration with the distal ends of each monomer embedded in the lipid membrane (Post et al., 1992;

Lindenbach and Rice, 1999). The E protein has both receptor binding (haemagglutin) and acid pH-dependent cell fusion activities, and composed of three structural domains. The third (domain III) contains a fold typical of an immunoglobulin constant domain and it is this domain that is thought to represent the cell receptor. There is considerable variation in amino acid sequence at the margins of this domain between tick- and mosquito-vectored flaviviruses. Some mutations in domain III equate with changes in virulence. In the case of yellow fever virus, there is one report that suggests a region of domain II may also be involved in binding virus to receptors present in monkey brains (Ni et al., 2000). Work on the structure of dengue virus E protein has progressed substantially over the past few years (see below) and comparative analyses should throw light on the detail of yellow fever receptor binding and substitutions to amino acids that equate to tissue tropism and attenuation.

Non-structural proteins

Despite the simplicity of protein expression, almost all of the non-structural proteins serve more than one function at some stage during the replication process. All seven are involved at various steps of RNA synthesis, although little is known as to how these interact with one another, and how each relates to those host proteins required for gene expression and RNA synthesis. The explosion of hepatitis C research, also a flavivirus, over the past 10 years has had a beneficial effect generally on our understanding of how flavivirus non-structural proteins function.

NS1 is an interesting protein, being glycosylated and essential for virus viability yet not found in the virus particle. It is translocated together with E protein into the lumen of the endoplasmic reticulum prior to cleavage at the E/NS1 junction by a host cell signalase. NS1 does not associate with mature virions, but locates in membrane-associated RNA complexes and thus promotes negative strand synthesis. In order to perform this function, NS1 combines with NS4A. Transcomplementation studies using NS1 deletion mutants of yellow fever virus and a replicon of Sindbis virus expressing the NS1 of dengue virus have shown that this interaction is virus specific, although variants of yellow fever virus have been detected that acquire recognition of dengue virus NS1 as a result of a single base change in the NS4A gene (Lindenbach and Rice, 1997, 1999).

NS1 can be detected both in and on the surface of infected cells, leading many workers to propose that NS1 could be the target of a CD8+ cytotoxic T cell response and a target for vaccine development. Jacobs et al. (2000) have suggested a role for NS1 as a cell activator as the addition of anti-NS1 antibody resulted in tyrosine phosphorylation of cellular proteins. NS1 is secreted by mammalian cells as a hexamer consisting of three homodimers. NS1 is not, however, secreted from infected mosquito cell lines (Smith and Wright, 1985). The extent of glycosylation and the processing of these sugar side chains contribute to the final structure of the resulting NS1 dimers. Variable glycosylation may also account for the difference in secretion properties of NS1 from mammalian and insect cells: one of the two polysaccharide side chains of the dengue virus NS1 is protected within the dimer from reaction with cellular glycosidases and remains high in mannose content, while the second remains exposed, being progressively trimmed and modified to form a multibranched endo-β-N-acetylglucosaminidase F resistant complex sugar (Flamand et al., 1999). Thus, complete processing of exposed, sugar side chains appears essential for NS1 secretion.

NS2A, NS2B, NS4A and NS4B collectively are a group of small hydrophobic proteins that facilitate the assembly of RNA replication complexes adjacent to cytoplasmic membranes. Neither of these gene products contains motifs homologous to other known mammalian or viral enzymes. Two forms of NS2A are known: one full length, the second with a truncated C-terminus. Mutations at the C-terminus of either form are lethal for yellow fever virus replication (Kummerer and Rice, 2002). The NS2B protein has two functional activities. First, NS2B combines with NS3 and acts as a co-factor for the NS3 serine protease. The second function utilises separate hydrophobic domains to facilitate the insertion of the NS2B–NS3 precursor into the endoplasmic reticulum at the time of translation. NS4A is not readily detected in a cleaved form within infected cells, being in the main part of a NS3–NS4A precursor. NS4B, in contrast, is readily seen, particularly in the perinuclear region. Late in the replication cycle NS4B can be found within the nucleus.

NS3 has two discrete functions. The first function is required for processing the polyprotein resulting from translation of the positive viral RNA strand. One-third of the N-terminal folds to form a serine protease. This part of the molecule contains motifs characteristic of the trypsin superfamily of proteases but in order to fulfil this proteolytic function prior coupling to NS2B is required, as mentioned above. Furthermore, efficient polyprotein processing requires binding to cellular membranes. The protease complex removes the anchor region from the C protein and recognises several other cleavage sites along the length of the polyprotein. All share a common motif consisting of two basic amino acids followed by an amino acid with a short side chain.

The heightened concern with regard to the increasing prevalence of persistent hepatitis C in the human population has stimulated work examining the NS3 protease of hepatitis C virus as a target for antivirals. This protein, along with other hepatitis C virus proteins, has now been analysed in considerable depth. The availability of structural co-ordinates allows for modelling of other NS3 proteins by threading and similar algorithms. Following this approach, a model of dengue NS3 has shown there are some differences in the substrate binding domain of the dengue virus NS3 protein (Brinkworth et al., 1999).

A fully functioning helicase is essential for flavivirus replication. The C-terminus contains regions homologous to the DEAD family of RNA helicases. The consensus is that the helicase plays a role in unwinding the secondary structure at the 3$'$ end of the viral positive strand template prior to the commencement of RNA synthesis, and perhaps also in releasing the nascent negative RNA strand prior to commencement of positive strand synthesis. NS3 also contains an RNA triphosphatase (NTPase) activity involved in the formation of the cap structure at the 5$'$ end of nascent positive RNA strands. This domain overlaps the protease activity between residues 160 and 180 of the dengue virus NS3 molecule (Li et al., 1999). NS3 interacts also with NS5, an interaction dependent on phosphorylation. The association with NS5 may regulate NS3 as NTPase activity is upregulated in its presence. The domains responsible for this interaction in dengue virus have been mapped to amino acids 320–368 on NS5, and 303–618 on NS3.

NS5 is the largest and most highly conserved of the non-structural proteins and constitutes the RNA-dependent RNA polymerase. Although with an overall basic charge, NS5 has long hydrophobic stretches that are more characteristic of a membrane-bound protein. The C-terminal portion contains the highly conserved GDD motif typical of viral RNA polymerases and protein modelling shows that NS5 structure resembles closely that of the poliovirus RNA polymerase. Other motifs along its length suggest that NS5 also has a role to play in the methylation of the $5'$ end cap structures. Both the methyltransferase function and the NS3-encoded triphosphatase represent two of the three enzymes necessary for $5'$ cap synthesis. A guanyltransferase would also be needed, but this activity has yet to be identified.

NS5 has been detected both in the cytoplasm and in the nucleus of infected cells. The nuclear form of NS5 is extensively phosphorylated. Translocation of NS5 into the nucleus is mediated by a nuclear localisation signal sited between the methyltransferase and polymerase domains. It is not known as what effect nuclear NS5 has on cellular functions, although differential phosphorylation of this protein during the replication cycle suggests nuclear-located NS5 has a role in the later stages of the replication cycle. Its presence in the nucleus may account for the basophilic staining bodies seen in infected cells. Current thinking is that cellular proteins complex with NS5 to direct and modulate RNA synthesis. Candidates for such proteins include the translation elongation factors EF-1, EF-Tu and EF-Ts. A further complexity is the reported interactions between NS5 and the nuclear transport receptor importin-β. These interactions can exclude NS3 from forming NS5–NS3 complexes, thus encouraging the migration of NS5 to the nucleus (Johansson et al., 2001).

Virus replication

The cellular receptor for yellow fever virus has yet to be defined although it is known that glycosaminoglycans play a role in virus entry. Two glycoprotein receptor molecules have been proposed for dengue 4 virus, and it may prove to be that entry requires more than one host component (Salas-Benito and del Angel, 1997). As flaviviruses also infect arthropod vectors, the cellular receptor for both mammalian cells and insect cells either has to be highly conserved or involve two separate domains.

Flavivirus particles enter the host cell by a process of receptor-mediated endocytosis followed by fusion at low pH of the viral envelope with the membrane of an endosomal vesicle. The nucleocapsid is then released into the cytoplasm. As most of the replication cycle takes place at or near the perinuclear membrane, there must be some mechanism of transporting the nucelocapsid through the cytoplasm, but at present this mechanism remains obscure.

Translation usually begins as a result of internal ribosome entry at the first AUG codon of the single open reading frame, although there is evidence of occasional initiation at the next AUG some 12–14 nucleotides downstream. After primary translation of the infecting viral genome, RNA synthesis begins by production of negative strand copies by the NS5 protein. Negative strand synthesis continues throughout the replication cycle. These negative copies are then used as templates for the generation of further positive RNA strands. RNA replication complexes are localised in the perinuclear endoplasmic reticulum and consist of both RNA double-stranded duplexes and replicative intermediates, the latter consisting of double-stranded regions and nascent single-stranded RNA molecules. These are either used as further plus strand templates or for translation. There are similarities here with poliovirus replication with the steady accumulation of structural proteins during the flavivirus replication cycle. This eventually leads to a point where nascent positive RNA strands are withdrawn from the pool of translatable plus strands to form new nucleocapsids. However, there seems to be a distinct compartmentalisation between polyprotein processing and RNA synthesis, and possibly moderated by such a topographical separation.

Hypertrophy and proliferation of cytoplasmic membranes are characteristic of flavivirus-infected cells. Nascent virus particles first assemble on the rough endoplasmic reticulum, and then these immature virions are transported progressively through the endoplasmic reticulum compartments to the cell surface where virus particles are released by exocytosis. Immediately prior to release the prM protein located within the viral envelope is cleaved by a host furin-type protease located in the trans-Golgi network. How this process occurs is difficult to analyse as visualisation of maturing yellow fever particles has proven difficult. Infected cells also release a non-infectious, subviral particle, for reasons that are unclear. These subviral particles are antigenic and represent cellular membrane fragments into which are inserted copies of the E and M proteins as well as small amounts of prM. As the E protein retains its haemagglutination properties, these particles are functionally referred to as the slowly sedimenting haemagglutinin (SHA) component.

Clinical disease

The clinical course of yellow fever develops through three distinct stages. The acute phase is characterised by a fever (39.5–40°C) of 3–4 days duration. Headache, back pain, nausea and vomiting constitute the major symptoms. At this stage, the patient is highly infectious with virus present in the blood from days 3–5. This viraemia ensures that the likelihood of human-to-human transmission by mosquitoes is high. Remission generally follows accompanied by a lowering of the fever. The headache disappears and the patient generally feels much recovered.

During the third stage, the fever returns with many if not all of the symptoms seen on presentation, but in a more severe form. The patient becomes increasingly anxious and agitated. Liver, heart and perhaps kidney failure follow rapidly accompanied by delirium. Jaundice is the inevitable result of the inflammation in the liver and death occurs 6–7 days after onset of the disease. Among those that survive, recovery can be slow. Virus cannot be recovered from the blood during this stage but anti-yellow fever virus antibodies can be detected, suggesting an immunopathological component late in the disease process.

During epidemics, the case fatality rate may exceed 50%, and for children can approach 70%, the major driver for the introduction of yellow fever vaccination into childhood immunisation programmes within endemic regions. In some outbreaks there has been a preponderance of males, for example the 1972–1973 outbreak in Brazil over 90% of cases were men. Despite suggestions to the contrary, there appears to be no link in disease severity according to ethnicity.

Other causes of viral haemorrhagic fever should always be suspected, such as Congo-Crimean haemorrhagic fever, Rift Valley fever, Marburg and Ebola viruses in Africa. Meningococcal septicaemia and leptospirosis are also infections that need to be eliminated during diagnosis.

Among other illnesses that can confound clinical diagnosis are the agents of viral hepatitis. Hepatitis A is common in endemic areas, indeed in Columbia and neighbouring countries hepatitis A is more common than other forms of viral hepatitis. Hepatitis A is rarely accompanied by a high fever, however, and serological tests for anti-hepatitis A IgM antibodies are readily available to differentiate this agent from yellow fever virus. The Rockefeller Foundation conducted surveillance measures in Brazil for many years based on the taking of liver tissue from fatal cases using a viscerotome. A re-examination by histopathology of samples taken between 1934 and 1967 has failed to show evidence of yellow fever antigens, however, although around 11% of the presumed yellow fever infections were positive for hepatitis B viral antigens (Simonetti et al., 2002), encouraging the speculation that these deaths may be more related to hepatitis B virus and its dependent agent hepatitis delta, the latter infection being particularly prevalent in the Amazonian basin.

Diagnosis

As with many virus infections, there is an emphasis on the detection of IgM antibodies during the early acute phase. The IgM capture ELISA is the test of preference, although care is needed with standardisation: cross-reactions do occur but can be minimised with care. Immunofluorescence using infected cells fixed previously in acetone is an easy method to adopt for field use and can be modified to detect either IgM or IgG antibodies, although the assay for IgG antibodies is sensitive to the presence of rheumatoid factor. A more definitive diagnosis is the presence of virus in the early viraemic period. Intracerebral or intraperitoneal inoculation of suckling mice is a sensitive method for virus detection but results may take up to 3 weeks. Intrathoracic inoculation of mosquitoes is also possible, but tissue culture isolation is perhaps preferable. Cell lines derived from either *Aedes albopictus* (C636 cells) or *Aedes pseudoscutellaris* (MOS61 cells) can readily support growth of yellow fever virus. Detection of virus replication by application of monoclonal antibodies can produce results in a few days. There is a risk that virus in samples is already complexed with antibodies thus dissociation of antigen–antibody complexes by treatment with the reducing agent dithiothreitol is recommended prior to inoculation of cell cultures.

Sequencing of yellow fever isolates has revealed that there are at least two, possibly three genotypes of yellow fever currently in circulation. Type I is found in Central and East Africa, type IIa in West Africa and type IIb in the Americas (Chang et al., 1995). These distinctions are based on phylogenetic analyses of the E protein. The relatively close association of strains from West Africa and the Americas is consistent with what we know of the historical origins of the virus in the New World, but it should be stressed that there are many phenotypic differences between isolates grouped in genotypes IIa and IIb. More needs to be done in defining to what extent such variation can result in virus adaptation to new hosts and mosquito vectors, and thus fundamentally alter the nature of the transmission cycle. Despite these differences, the presently available yellow fever vaccines protect against all three genotypes.

Pathology

The taking of a liver biopsy is not advisable given the high risk of haemorrhage. However, liver tissue taken at autopsy is useful for epidemiological purposes, as mentioned above. The hepatitis associated with yellow fever virus is manifested by the presence of extensive mid-zonal necrosis, visceral haemorrhages, sinusoidal acidophilic bodies and hypertrophy of Kupffer cells. The portal tracts become extensively infiltrated with monocytes. Histopathology shows the appearance of dark eosinophilic bodies in the cytoplasm of hepatocytes (Councilman bodies) (Fig. 5). These remnants of hepatocytes having undergone apopotosis were often regarded as specific to yellow fever but caution needs to be exercised as similar inclusions can be due to other causes of viral haemorrhagic disease.

Prevention and control

Yellow fever vaccines owe their origins to work carried out in the 1920s and early 1930s under the sponsorship of the Rockefeller Foundation. In 1928 it was found that monkeys were susceptible to yellow fever virus, an observation that led directly to the isolation of Asibi strain of yellow fever virus from present-day Ghana together with the Dakar strain obtained from a Senegalese patient. Shortly after, Theiler discovered that Swiss white

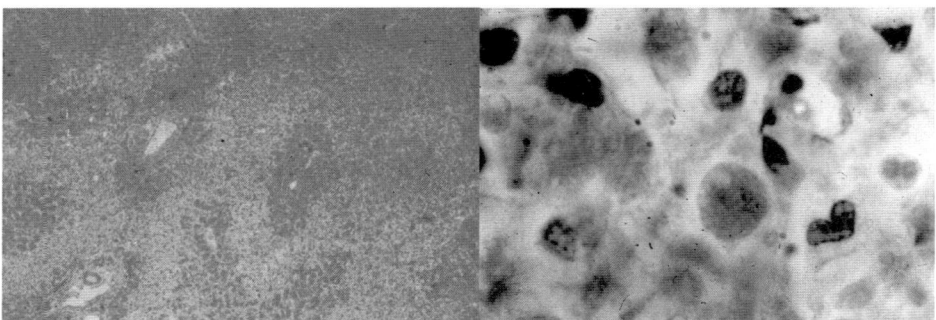

Fig. 5 Histopathological examination of liver parenchyma from a patient showing inflammation around the portal tracts (arrowed; a) and the distinctive presence of Councilman bodies (b).

mice could also be infected, thus opening up a method for measuring neutralising antibodies.

Two live attenuated vaccines were developed concurrently using these isolates. French workers passaged the Dakar isolate 128 times in mice brains to derive what became known as the French neurotropic vaccine. This product was used in the Francophile community for some years at the 258–260 passage level but its use was discontinued owing to systemic reactions in up to 20% of those vaccinated. The second vaccine lineage was derived from the Asibi strain. Present day vaccines all have their origin in this virus originally recovered in West Africa. It is important to note that both the French neurotropic vaccine and the 17D strains have lost both the capacity to produce viscerotropic disease and an ability to replicate in mosquitoes.

The 17D vaccine strains were originally developed by Theiler and colleagues by passage first in mouse brain and then in chick embryo tissue. Two substrains of the 17D attenuated virus form the basis of present vaccines. The first is based upon virus derived at the 204th passage (17D-204) and is used predominantly in Europe and Africa at the 234–238 passage level. The second originates from the 195th passage of the lineage, being subsequently passaged independently in embryonated eggs and used at the 286–288 passage level (17DD): this is used almost exclusively in South America. Thus, there is a dichotomy in passage history between vaccines used in the Americas and the Old World (Fig. 6). Although differing in lineage, both are equally effective, despite evidence of phenotypic differences between yellow fever virus circulating in the Americas and Africa.

Protection against yellow fever—indeed against any human flavivirus infection—is mediated by the presence of neutralising antibodies. Seroconversion rates in healthy recipients rise to over 95% by 30 days following a single dose of live attenuated vaccine. Immunity is probably lifelong although revaccination after 10 years is required under the International Health Regulations. The vaccine is delivered subcutaneously and is well tolerated. It can be given simultaneously with other live attenuated vaccines such as measles and polio as well as together with DPT, oral cholera, typhoid, hepatitis A and hepatitis B vaccines. Mild adverse reactions are experienced by up to 25% of recipients, these generally lasting a few days and consist of pain and soreness at the site of injection, headache, malaise and myalgia.

The vaccine is contraindicated for pregnant women unless demanded by local circumstances. Inadvertent vaccination in early pregnancy can lead to anxiety, but a study by Robert et al. (1999) suggested that inadvertent exposure in the first trimester does not increase the risk of abnormalities during gestation. There is no evidence of the vaccine crossing the placenta. A study by Nasidi et al. (1993) among 40 Nigerian women and their offspring showed no evidence of congenital infection despite vaccination during pregnancy. Seroconversion was less than 40% as opposed to more than 85% among the general population, suggesting that immunosuppression during pregnancy suppressed the B cell response to the 17D virus.

The issue of immunosuppression in patients with HIV and responsiveness to yellow fever vaccine has not been sufficiently investigated. The expectation is that such individuals would not respond as well as others and could be more susceptible

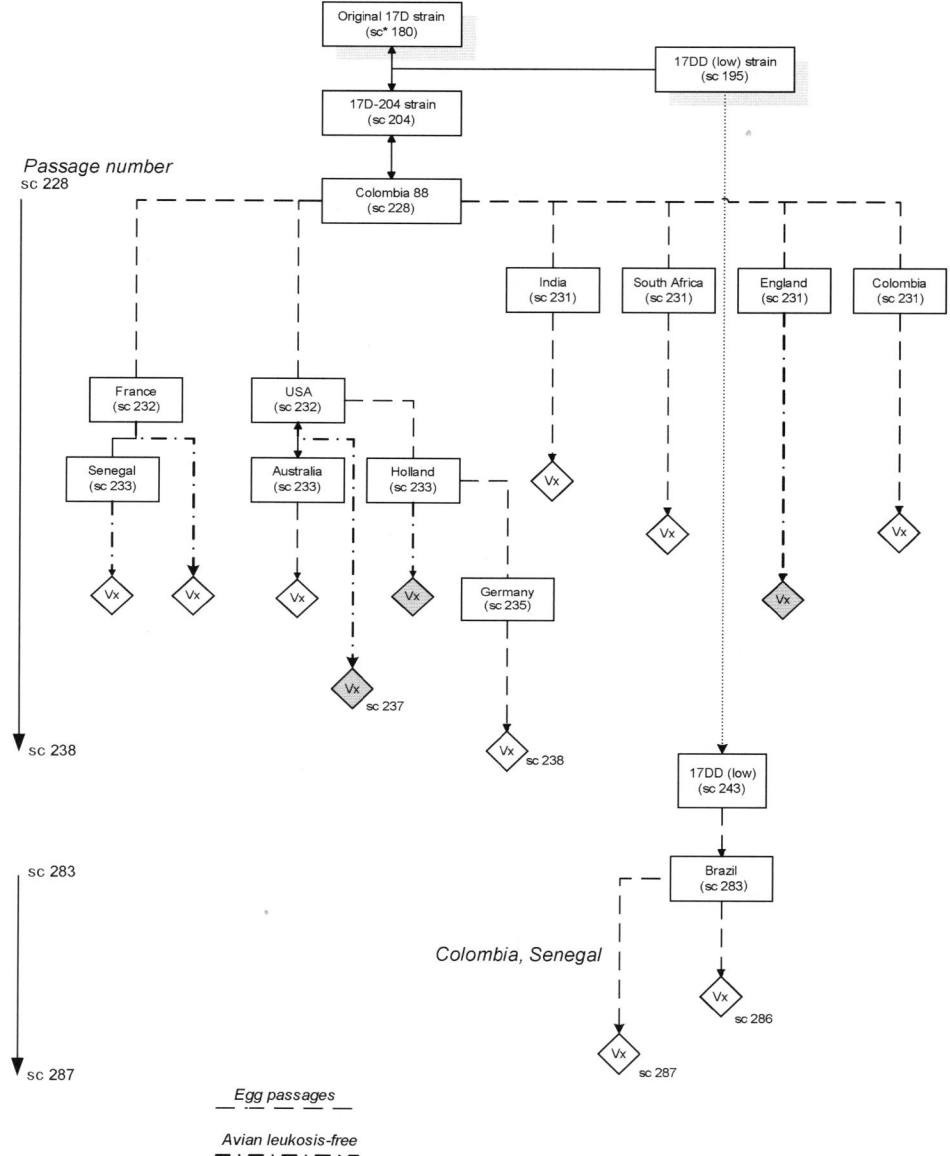

Fig. 6 Lineage of currently licensed yellow fever (17D) vaccine strains.

to the consequences of infection, but this hypothesis has not been tested. As the vaccine is produced in eggs, residual egg protein may prove difficult in those with allergies to eggs but again this has not been borne out in practice, with allergic reactions being as infrequent as one per million of individuals vaccinated.

The viraemia following vaccination is low, normally below $2 \log_{10}$ pfu, and is of short duration. Thus, the risk of vaccine virus transmission by insect bite is low, but in any event the 17D virus is substantially attenuated to the extent that it is unable to replicate in mosquito vectors.

Presently vaccine continues to be manufactured in embryonated chicken eggs. Attempts to replace the egg-derived products with virus grown in cell monolayers such as chick fibroblasts have been frustrated by the low yields that result from infection of cell cultures with the 17D virus. There is also the question of cost. Egg-grown virus is cheap to produce and the technology readily transposed into endemic areas where investment in expensive cell culture facilities is limited and skilled personnel rarely available. Some embryonated hens' eggs are contaminated with avian leucosis virus; although there is no evidence to suggest the presence of this contaminant has any effect on efficacy or the health of vaccines, it is thought desirable to eliminate this agent from yellow fever vaccine products. A WHO-approved master seed lot free of ALV has been available from the Robert Koch Institute in Berlin for some years but as yet has not been universally adopted.

The long history in the use of the 17D substrains presents a unique opportunity to define the molecular basis of attenuation and obtain indicators as to how vaccines could be developed against dengue and other flaviviruses, particularly vaccines against those infections that as yet have proved too difficult to develop for various reasons.

The genome of yellow fever virus was first sequenced using 17D-204 virus held by the American Type Culture Collection (Rice et al., 1985). This landmark study has since been followed by completing the sequence of both the wild type Asibi virus as originally isolated by Stoker and the complementary 17DD virus subjected to an independent lineage beyond passage 195 in chick embryos. These studies together with related work have revealed a number of differences at the molecular level: for example, there are 32 amino acid differences between the Asibi isolate and the 17D-204 virus distributed throughout the structural and non-structural proteins with most variation in the E and NS2A proteins. Four nucleotide substitutions in the $3'$ non-coding region are found consistently in all vaccine strains, and the nucleotide sequence in the $5'$ non-coding region (NTR) is highly conserved. Parallel studies of the Dakar isolate and its derived French Neurotropic vaccine strain have similarly demonstrated a proportionally high mutation rate in the E and NS2A proteins (Wang et al., 1995), but with little concordance in the nature of individual substitutions. Only two substitutions are common: a leucine to phenylalanine change in M protein at position 36, and an isoleucine to methionine change at position 95 in NS4B. The fact that monoclonal antibody studies show cross-reactivity for viruses with dissimilar linear amino acid sequences indicates the importance of conformational epitopes in eliciting neutralising antibodies. Interestingly, the 17DD strain possesses an additional glycosylation site on the E protein at position 153 not present on 17D-204 virus, and the new master seed lot approved by WHO possesses a new glycosylation site close by at position 151. The significance of such differences is unclear but could affect either the conformation of a critical determinant or its immunogenicity.

An important issue is the potential of vaccine strains to revert to neurovirulence. There have been a handful of cases reported in vaccines, mainly in children less than 1 year of age. Only one fatal case has been reported: a 3-year-old girl who was immunised with the 17D-204 virus (Jennings et al., 1994). This case is notable as virus was reisolated from the child and subjected to antigenic analysis, showing that the virus had regained reactivity for a monoclonal antibody normally reactive only with wild type virus. The isolate was also neurovirulent for a single cynomolgus monkey. Sequencing of this isolate has shown a number of mutations (Barrett, 1997). Interestingly one of the changes was at position 155 on the E protein, close to the glycosylation site discussed above. Notwithstanding this and rare instances of encephalitis in vaccinees, it needs to be stressed that yellow fever vaccination remains one of the greatest medical achievements in the control of infectious diseases.

The experience of over 60 years of routine use has provided substantial evidence that the 17D virus is both safe and highly efficacious. For this reason, the 17D vaccine strain makes an ideal candidate for use as a live vector for genes of other, heterologous antigens, most notably for genes coding for the structural proteins of other flaviviruses, such as hepatitis C, dengue and West Nile viruses. Studies using chimeric yellow fever—dengue constructs are described later in this chapter. This platform technology owes its origins to the work of Pletnev et al. (1992) who showed the potential of a chimeric virus containing genes from tick-borne encephalitis virus and Japanese encephalitis virus as a human vaccine. This work established the important principle that the chimera construct had lost peripheral invasiveness as a result of the vector construction.

Dengue

Colonisation of the New World brought with it infections previously unknown to the indigenous populations of the Americas. These included smallpox, measles, scarlet fever, malaria and yellow fever. It is probable that cases of the latter could have well been mistaken for dengue fever as examination of historical records makes it impossible to distinguish the two infections apart until at least the end of the 18th century. Between 1779 and 1780 detailed descriptions were made of outbreaks resembling present-day dengue fever from the nascent United States, Africa and the Dutch East Indies. The most celebrated of these descriptions is due to Benjamin Rush, a physician of Philadelphia and a close friend and colleague of the American Founding Fathers (Fig. 1).

Rush is generally credited as being the first to provide a detailed description of what we now know as dengue fever. This was largely based on an outbreak occurred in Philadelphia in the summer of 1780 which Rush described as a bilious remittent fever. The description has remained little improved over the centuries, so fastidious was Rush in ensuring he committed to record an accurate and objective observation as to the course of the disease. His descriptions were all the more remarkable given that a number of illnesses were circulating in Philadelphia at that time. Although he did not to make the connection with a possible vector, he noted that "…mosquitoes were uncommonly numerous during the autumn" (quoted in Humphreys, 1997). That he failed to make the connection is all the more remarkable given that Rush recorded the epidemic as subsiding as soon as the temperature dropped sharply in October. The locals referred to the malady as "breakbone fever". Coincidentally Rush was also renowned for his interest in mental disorders, and records the case of two afflicted sisters, both of whom suffered from dejection and depression, pressed Rush to change the name to "breakheart fever".

Concurrently David Bylon, a physician in the Dutch East Indies noted a similar disease which he referred to as *knokkel-koorts* ("Knuckle fever"). Humphreys has pointed out that the prominence of knuckle pain means this could have been an outbreak of Chikungunya virus, not breakbone fever as was supposed by his contemporaries. The name dengue came into use after reports of an outbreak in the Spanish West Indies between 1827 and 1828 when the Swahili term *Ki denga pepo* was first used to describe the disease.

Dengue fever epidemics in the 18th and 19th centuries occurred in the Americas and elsewhere in regular cycles, reflecting the fact that transport by sea took many weeks, if not months, between Europe and the newly emerging empires of the Netherlands and Britain. The rapid changes of the 20th century changed dramatically the epidemiology of dengue virus, especially the upheavals accompanying the Second World War and its aftermath. It was at this time that the first extensively documented outbreak of dengue haemorrhagic fever (DHF) occurred in the Philippines in 1953. This was followed 5 years later by a much larger outbreak in Thailand. Since the 1960s dengue has spread to over 60 countries, with extensive epidemics particularly in the Caribbean and South America. Although outbreaks are known to occur in Africa, less is known about these, most likely because if and when they do occur the infrastructure for reporting such outbreaks is invariably poor.

Although dengue fever as an acute illness has a low mortality rate, its impact, like that of yellow fever, extends beyond its clinical importance. In centuries past, the introduction of infection into a community could mean economic disaster for fledgling colonies. In modern times, the impact of an infectious disease such as dengue can still result in serious economic loss in a country heavily dependent upon tourism. For example, Puerto Rico was hit by a devastating epidemic in 1979 that resulted in a loss of over $10 million, made far worse by dengue returning no less than eight times with losses amounting eventually to over $100 million. The 1981 outbreak in Cuba had a similar devastating impact, with a further economic cost of approximately $100 million. The four serotypes of dengue virus extend over regions inhabited by over 2.5 billion people, i.e. over a third of the human population are at risk. This makes dengue arguably the most important of virus diseases spread by arthropods.

Epidemiology

Dengue viruses are transmitted to humans by the bite of an infected female *Aedes* mosquito. The principal vector is *A. aegypti*, a black and white mosquito that has become highly adapted to an urban environment. The female needs regular blood meals in order to provide nutrients for its eggs, which it lays in containers of still water commonly found close to domestic dwellings, for example open water barrels, flower pots and old tins and containers. Old car tyres provide ideal vessels for still water and at least one outbreak in Taiwan has been attributed to *Aedes* larvae imported in a cargo of recycled tyres. The adults are difficult to detect, feeding off humans in daylight, with bites often going unnoticed. Civic programmes aimed at eliminating the vector by removing open containers of still water have done much to reduce, if not entirely eliminate, the risk of transmission in urban areas. These measures are often backed by the force of law as in the case of Singapore, for example.

A. *aegypti* has a worldwide distribution in the tropical zones, but for reasons unknown dengue is not always found in regions infested with this replication-competent vector. Epidemics first occurred in the 1950s in South East Asia and over the ensuring 30 years spread first through the Philippines to the South Pacific islands, and from there spread to Central and South America, parts of Africa, India and south to Queensland in Australia. Dengue viruses have a considerable propensity to spread further, particularly as A. *aegypti* has returned to many areas since the cessation of insecticide spraying. The disease threatens the southern United States, the populous areas of Brazil and could spread to much of Africa (Fig. 7).

Once a female mosquito imbibes blood from a viraemic human, the virus replicates in the gut of the insect, moving to the salivary glands by 8–11 days after ingestion. The female mosquito remains infected for life, transmitting virus in its saliva each time the insect acquires a new blood meal. A. *albopictus*, the tiger mosquito—so named owing to its aggressive behaviour—is also replication competent. This species has recently invaded the southern USA, setting the stage for possible future outbreaks.

Although A. *aegypti* is responsible for human-to-human transmission in an urban environment, a sylvatic cycle has increasingly been recognised, at least in Asia.

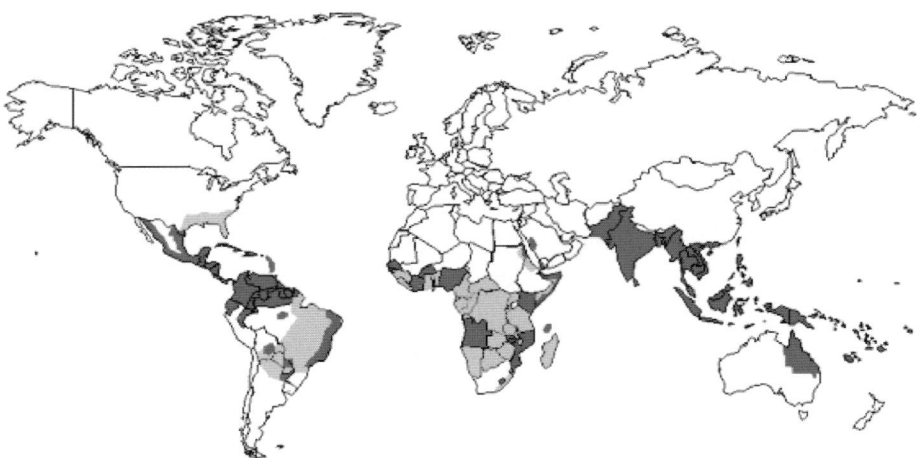

Fig. 7 Geographical distribution of *Aedes aegypti* and dengue virus. The denser the shade, the greater the incidence of disease (courtesy of the World Health Organisation).

Forest-dwelling mosquitoes of the genus *Ochlerotatus* transmit the virus between monkeys—principally *Macaca* and *Presbytis* species. This cycle is likely complex as *A. albopictus* can also transmit the virus at the edge of forested areas. In Africa, *Erythrocebus* monkeys are the principal hosts in the rain forests, with other Aedine mosquitoes also contributing to maintenance of the transmission cycle, for example *A. luteocephalus*, *A. taylor-furcifer* and *A. opok* (Gubler, 1998; Wang et al., 2000). There is evidence of all four serotypes of dengue virus[3] originating in monkeys, with adaptation to humans having occurred both relatively recently and independently for all four serotypes. Although the sylvatic cycle has been demonstrated for all four serotypes in Asia, only a dengue 2 sylvatic cycle has been demonstrated in Africa (Rodhain, 1991). Understanding more regarding the sylvatic cycle would boost our understanding of genetic variation between and within the four virus serotypes: dengue virus has evolved to the extent that it is not dependent upon the enzootic cycle for persistence in any given geographical locality.

Clinical features

Seroprevalence studies have shown that the majority of dengue virus infections are asymptomatic. Clinical disease is of two distinct types. The first is dengue fever, the "classical" disease seen in the vast majority of cases among adults who have not been previously exposed to the virus. The second is the haemorrhagic form of the disease, DHF, which may or may not progress to dengue shock syndrome (DSS).

Classical dengue fever is characterised by a sudden rise in body temperature, accompanied by nausea and a severe headache, the latter most often located towards the frontal regions and accompanied by retro-orbital pain. Other neurological signs include severe depression, apathy and complaints of disturbing dreams. However, the most distinctive feature is the severe muscle and bone pain, particularly in the lower back. Joint pains, a lymphadenopathy and vomiting all develop over the next 3–7 days. A diffuse and discrete macropapaular rash develops immediately prior to recovery. Although incapacitating, the acute illness is relatively short lived and patients eventually make a full recovery although many remain incapacitated for many weeks during convalescence.

The more severe disease of DHF is seen in children below the age of 15 and in those infected previously with dengue virus. Clinically, DHF resembles yellow fever in that the initial stages of the disease—similar to uncomplicated dengue fever—is followed by a brief respite when body temperature returns to near normal, only to be followed by a sharp onset of fever once more and a rapid deterioration in the patient's condition. The patient displays profound prostration and shows progressively all the manifestations of haemorrhage and shock that result from circulatory collapse and hypotension. The liver may become enlarged with signs of jaundice. Petechiae appear in the skin and patients give a positive tourniquet test. Ecchymoses, gastrointestinal bleeding and haemorrhagic pneumonia become evident.

---

[3] By convention, the four serotypes are frequently referred to as DEN-1, DEN-2, DEN-3 and DEN-4, respectively.

Table 1

WHO classification of dengue haemorrhagic fever

Grade	Clinical description
I	Fever with non-specific, constitutional symptoms and the only haemorrhagic manifestations being a positive tourniquet test
II	As for Grade I, but accompanied by more extensive haemorrhagic manifestations
III	Signs of circulatory failure or hypertension
IV	Profound shock with pulse and blood pressure being undetectable (DSS)

The World Health Organisation has attempted to produce a case definition of DHF as a sudden febrile onset accompanied by haemorrhagic manifestations that include a positive tourniquet test and an increase in haematocrit reading to 20% or more. This case definition has been the subject of much debate, with many experts emphasising that the disease profile differs according to the age of the patient and geographical location. In order to aid the collation of clinical data, the WHO has proposed classifying DHF in four grades (Table 1).

Although severe muscle and bone pain together with a sudden onset of fever are highly suggestive of dengue fever, the disease on presentation may resemble many other febrile illnesses. The more severe form, DHF, may be confused clinically with other causes of haemorrhagic disease, although haemoconcentration and indications of a coagulopathy may be useful in pointing towards dengue virus as a cause.

Although the risk of DHF and DSS increases significantly with secondary infections, the risk does not increase further on a subsequent third exposure to another serotype. If anything, the risk appears to decline, perhaps as a result of previous infection stimulating a sufficiently broad immune response that replication by a third serotype is contained.

Diagnosis

In contrast to most flaviviruses that cause human disease, virus isolation can prove difficult from cases of dengue fever. Direct intracerebral injection into suckling mice often requires several blind passages for an isolate to become evident. An alternative approach is the intracerebral inoculation of *Toxorhynchites* ticks, with successful isolation possible in less than 3 days. Intrathoracic inoculation of mosquitoes is another possibility, with isolation taking somewhat longer at up to a week. Virus isolation in cell culture is to be preferred, however. Insect cell lines are very sensitive to dengue virus: the most widely available is the C6-36 cell line derived from *A. albopictus*, but alternatives are AP-61 cells from *A. pseudoscutellaris* and TRA-248 cells from the tick *Toxorhynchites ambionensis*. Regular inspection of replicate cultures by addition of fluorescent- or peroxidase-labelled monoclonal antibody specific for dengue virus usually produces a positive response within 3 days of inoculation.

Specific serology is vital to making an accurate diagnosis. ELISA assays designed to detect IgM are increasingly replacing haemagglutinin inhibition for the detection of anti-dengue virus antibodies. IgM antibodies are present from as early as the third day of infection and may persist for as long as 3 months. Rapid tests for IgG antibodies are common, but care needs to be taken to ensure that tests are adequately controlled for unwanted cross-reactions with other flaviviruses. Immunofluorescence is useful as each visual field contains a number of uninfected cells that can serve as negative controls. The complement-fixation test has now largely fallen out of use, mainly because of its complexity, its relative insensitivity compared to other methods, and the difficulties in standardising reagents. Tests for measuring neutralising antibodies are particularly useful in confirming both the diagnosis and for determining the serotype of an isolate.

Properties of dengue virus

The dengue virus genome is a single-stranded RNA molecule of positive sense with respect to gene expression. Approximately 11 kb in length, the genome organisation is similar to that of yellow fever virus (see Fig. 4).

Electron microscopy of extracellular virus shows a particle of approximately 50 nm in diameter with clearly visible surface projections. The core protein exists in an ordered structure less well defined compared to that of the alphaviruses, where the core assumes an icosahedral symmetry dictated by the envelope glycoproteins as the virus buds from an infected cell, a process mediated by interactions with the alphavirus E2 envelope glycoprotein. Such interactions appear to be absent in dengue and other flaviviruses.

Knowledge of the three-dimensional structure is important for identifying regions that can be targeted to block virus entry and for designing new vaccines, as well as elucidating just how heterologous neutralising antibodies can cause antibody-mediated enhancement. Most flaviviruses have around 40% identical amino acids in their E proteins, and thus the overall three-dimensional structure in terms of secondary structure elements such as folds and management of functional domains is likely to be similar. The structure of the tick-borne encephalitis virus E protein was determined in 1995 (Rey et al., 1995) but despite the increasing sophistication of modelling methods standard alignment methods proved insufficient to predict the secondary structure of the remaining 60% of the dengue virus E protein.

The class II fusion (E) protein of dengue virus has a distinctly different structure to the class I fusion protein of the haemagglutinin of influenza virus. In common with the E protein of tick-borne encephalitis virus, the dengue E protein is ordered as 90 dimers flat-packed on the surface of an icosahedral-shaped virus particle. The dimers are so closely packed on the surface of dengue virus that the viral membrane is inaccessible at physiological pH and thus fusion cannot occur. Reducing the pH results in a conformational change, resulting in the dimers re-arranging to form a $T = 3$ icosahedral lattice (Kuhn et al., 2002). The net effect is an increase in particle diameter and the exposure of the underlying viral membrane.

The E protein is not cleaved during the maturation and assembly of new virus and is predominately non-helical, being composed largely of β-sheets. Each monomer is orientated in an opposite head-to-tail arrangement with respect to its partner, and structural studies show there are three distinct domains. Domains I and III are located at either ends of the dimer and opposite the complementary domain on the other monomer. Domain II is an elongated, finger-like structure with a hydrophobic sequence (approximating to residues 98–109 for the dengue 2 virus E protein) conserved between all of the flaviviruses. It is this region that is responsible for interacting with the host cell membranes following uptake of virus into endosomes and performs a function analogous to that of the N-terminal domain of class I fusion proteins such as the haemagglutinin molecule of influenza virus (see below).

Recently the structure of the dengue E protein has yielded to X-ray crystallography, illustrating that E protein contains a binding pocket for a hydrophobic ligand (Modis et al., 2003). Binding to a lipid on the target cell is thought to trigger a conformational change in E which presages membrane fusion. The presence of mannose appears important for receptor binding (Hung et al., 1999). There are two putative N-linked glycosylation sites: the first (ASN-153) is highly conserved among flaviviruses whereas the second (ASN-67) is specific for dengue virus. Virus replication in mosquito cells results in the addition of sugars to both asparagine residues and these play a role in identifying the C-type lectin DC-SIGN that is present on the surface of human dendritic cells (Navarro-Sanchez et al., 2003).

A number of cellular ligands have been suggested as forming the receptor for E. These include heparin sulphate (Chen et al., 1997), CD-14 (Chen et al., 1999) and a variety of glycoproteins (Marianneau et al., 1996; Hung et al., 1999). However, these are absent on the surface of dendritic cells that support virus replication. Moreover, immature dendritic cells appear more susceptible to virus than mature DCs (Wu et al., 2000). These cells express DC-SIGN, a C-type lectin that has been implicated in the susceptibility of dendritic cells to a spectrum of viruses, including Ebola (Alvarez et al., 2002). Tassaneetrithep et al. (2003) have shown that THP-1 cells transfected with DC-SIGN become susceptible to dengue and infectious particles can be recovered from culture supernatants. DC-SIGN has an homology with L-SIGN present on endothelial cells, and thus a similar interaction between virus and the epithelium may be instrumental in triggering the vascular changes that are a feature of dengue pathogenesis.

Cell fusion plays a role in initiating dengue and other flavivirus infections. Most of our knowledge as to how membrane fusion occurs has been obtained by studies in influenza virus, where fusion is initiated by a trimeric structure consisting of a coiled coil helix immediately adjacent to the fusion peptide. The latter is inserted into the host cell membrane, leading to the formation of a six-bundle helix (Skehel and Wiley, 1998). Stretches of hydrophobic amino acids make up the fusion peptide: these adapt either helices (associated with class I fusion events) and β barrels (class II fusion). Both allow charged (polar) amino acid side chains to become internalised, with hydrophobic exteriors promoting insertion amongst the aliphatic chains of a lipid bilayer.

The mechanism of these interactions has been clarified by Modis et al. (2004). After a lowering of pH within the endosome, the structure undergoes a substantial change in structure. The re-organisation of dimers into trimers results in the domain II fusion loops forming projections approximately 100 Å in length, the hydrophobic tips being inserted into the host membrane. The outer surface of the trimer contains grooves with the potential to interact with the anchor regions (domain III): these domains rotate during the fusion process, thus promoting distortion of the viral and host membranes leading to an irreversible conformational change and providing the necessary energy for fusion. The major significance of having class II structures would be one of speed (Corver et al., 2000). In the case of the class I structures of orthomyxoviruses, there is a prior requirement for the release of a fusion peptide and multiple interactions between subunits before fusion can occur. These reorganisations take longer than is probably the case for class II-mediated fusion where the envelope proteins are already ordered on the virus surface.

Phylogenetic analyses and evolution

Dengue virus is divisible into four distinct serotypes using conventional plaque-reduction neutralisation assays (Russell and Nisalak, 1967). The four serotypes may differ by as much as 40% in amino acid sequence of the envelope (E) protein which bears the ligand for neutralising antibodies. Dengue 1 and dengue 3 are the most closely related, with dengue 2 being somewhat more distant and dengue 4 virus the most divergent. Although it is possible that all four serotypes may have evolved in geographically isolated regions, today all four co-circulate in many areas of Africa, Asia and the Americas. Within each serotype, however, there does not appear to be much antigenic drift, which bodes well for vaccine development once the major obstacles of producing a polyvalent vaccine are overcome (see below).

The recent use of comparative gene analysis has stimulated work into defining the origin of dengue virus serotypes, and how the virus has evolved in association with its primate hosts. In particular, dengue virus is a paradigm of virus evolution in response to changing host numbers, immunity, behaviour and environment. Zanotto et al. (1996) compared the rate of nucleotide substitution between 123 mosquito- and tick-borne flavivirus genome sequences and concluded that those flaviviruses dependent upon mosquitoes for transmission evolve at around twice the rate of tick-borne viruses. Vector biology may account for at least some of this difference. The data discussed by Zanotto and colleagues suggests that, although dengue and yellow fever may have diverged more than 3000 years ago, the rate of evolution has not been constant, and that it is only in the last two centuries that dengue has undergone rapid divergence into four serotypes that are so distinct as no longer showing properties of serological cross-neutralisation. This accelerated divergence has paralleled the exponential increase in the global human population since the late 18th century when dengue first became apparent. The argument is that individual communities need to reach a certain size in order to sustain any new emerging variants.

Pathogenesis

The question as to why only a minority of patients develop DHF and DSS whilst the vast majority of cases do not is one of the biggest challenges of dengue research. Hypotheses abound, but the two main hypotheses are those focusing on variability of the virus and the role of the host immune response, particularly antibodies. Against this background there are clear epidemiological differences from region to region that implies host susceptibility may also be important in determining disease outcome.

Strain variability

There is some evidence that virus variability may be a determining factor. Originally expounded by Rosen and colleagues over 30 years ago, this hypothesis states that virulence and disease outcome is determined by the genetic properties of the virus, the more virulent strains giving rise to the sequelae of DHF and DSS. Since this hypothesis was first proposed, there has been much debate as to whether certain strains can be linked to disease severity. The rapid advance in sequencing technology has added a further dimension to the somewhat anecdotal evidence of the past that has relied exclusively on serology. Perhaps the most convincing evidence that genotypic variation may be important stems from the observation that the so-called "American" strain of dengue 2 virus is not associated with DHF and DSS. This "American" genotype was responsible for an outbreak centred on Iquitos in Peru in 1995 (Watts et al., 1999). Over 50,000 secondary infections are known to have occurred but remarkably not a single case of DHF or DSS was seen. By comparison, in South East Asia at least 900 cases would have been expected during an outbreak of this size. In contrast, a dengue 2 virus outbreak in Cuba 14 years earlier—due to a different genotype —resulted in over 300,000 infections with 30,000 instances of illness progressing to DHF and DSS.

The relative avirulence of the "American" dengue 2 virus genotype has been attributed to an amino acid substitution at reside 390 of the envelope (E) glycoprotein, a change that certainly reduces the ability of the virus to replicate in cultures of monocyte-derived macrophages (Pryor et al., 2001). It is most unlikely that this is the sole explanation, however, as Shurtleff et al. (2001) showed that an American genotype strain was responsible for an outbreak in Venezuela characterised by a significant number of cases progressing to DHF and DSS. It is possible that the lack of DHF/DSS cases in Peru in 1991 was due to pre-existing antibodies to dengue 1 virus (Kochel et al., 2002). Antibody affinity may also be an important factor as well as antibody specificity. Also the length of time that elapsed from previous exposure to the heterologous serotype will determine the titre of residual reactive antibodies in patients suffering secondary infections and their capacity to complex with infectious virus. Nothing is known regarding immunological memory to these antigenic components, nor the extent to which a secondary antibody response can be triggered to the second virus.

Perhaps more critical in undermining this hypothesis is the failure to find significant sequence variation between dengue virus isolates taken from cases of acute dengue fever and those with the more severe DHF illness presenting at the same time and in the same locality (Rico-Hesse et al., 1997, 1998; Uzcategui et al., 2001). In addition, many of these studies have lacked data as to viral load, an important factor in determining just how readily virus can be transmitted via insect bite between humans. There is some evidence associating disease severity with viral burden (Vaughn et al., 2000) and certainly in other diseases such as Lassa fever and hepatitis C viral load can be an important marker of disease progression.

The role of antibody

Antibody-mediated enhancement has been shown for a number of virus infections, for example rabies and HIV, thus this is not a phenomenon restricted to dengue virus. A significant number of cases have been recorded in patients with pre-existing IgG antibodies to at least one of the other four serotypes of dengue virus. Halstead and O'Rourke (1977) proposed that such pre-existing antibodies complexed with infectious virus introduced during a subsequent infection with a heterologous virus: the resulting immune complexes result in a much greater uptake of infectious virus into susceptible cells expressing Fc receptors for antibody on their surface, such as macrophages. There is some experimental support for this hypothesis. Heterologous antibody can enhance the uptake of virus into cultured macrophages and the infection *in vivo* is more severe in rhesus monkeys injected with virus complexed with heterologous antibodies, whether these be from hyperimmune antisera or human sera. There is strong epidemiological and clinical support for this concept from work in South East Asia where DHF occurs predominantly in children. Pre-existing antibodies can be acquired from their mothers during the first year of life or in older infants and children as a result of a previous infection. In the Cuban epidemic of 1981, DHF occurred mainly in children exposed to dengue 1 virus 4 years previously when up to several million individuals were likely exposed to the virus.

There is every possibility that these findings cannot be so readily extended to understanding the pathogenesis of severe dengue infection in the Americas and elsewhere. Notwithstanding this caveat, most workers agree that antibody-mediated enhancement of virus uptake does play some role in dengue virus pathogenesis, but that it is unlikely to be the sole explanation as to why some cases progress to DHF and DSS. One of the major unknowns is just how variable an antigenic domain needs to be before a complexed antibody will fail to neutralise infectivity but still bind with sufficient affinity to allow the infectious virus–antibody complex to be taken up by susceptible cells. There have been some inroads to our understanding of the immune mechanisms that may be at work in such patients (for a review, see Kurane and Takasaki, 2001).

Host susceptibility

As with many human illnesses, there is always a suggestion that disease progression may be linked to the HLA type of the host (Chiewsilp et al., 1981; Stephens et al., 2002). This is reminiscent of attempts to link persistent hepatitis C and HIV with HLA haplotype, but studies with dengue virus often lack statistical power to offer any meaningful conclusions. T cell activation is linked to cells bearing V-β-17, but there does not appear to be any evidence of a "superantigen" effect. What is clear is that age at the time of exposure is important, together with sex and whether or not the person has had any previous exposure to dengue virus.

Treatment

Management of DHF and DSS is limited to supportive therapy. Symptoms can be alleviated by administering analgesics and aspirin to bring down the fever. Intravenous fluids counter fluid loss, especially when haemorrhage is present and the patient shows signs of shock. The administration of blood products is often considered.

Public health and the control of dengue

The impact of dengue on human health in affected countries is considerable. Apart from the obvious distress to infected persons, the economic burden is high, accounted largely by the additional medical care required, the need to implement expensive programmes of mosquito eradication and the indirect consequences on service industries increasingly dependent upon tourism. At present neither dengue nor yellow fever is a serious public health threat to countries outside of endemic areas but habitat areas supporting mosquitoes capable of transmitting dengue virus have rapidly expanded, becoming well established in the southern states of the USA and in Southern Europe.

A number of factors account for the spread and upsurge in dengue virus over the last 30–40 years. These are summarised in Table 2. First, major demographic changes have taken place, particularly in Asia and on the Indian subcontinent. A rapid increase in birth rate combined with a steady migration of rural populations into major conurbations has resulted in extensive proliferation of shantytowns and other areas with sub-standard sanitary conditions. These conditions are ideal for the spread of infectious diseases, including those dependent upon arthropod vectors. Modern society makes abundant use of plastic and polystyrene containers which when carelessly discarded adds to the already numerous nooks and crannies in which mosquito larvae can develop.

The rise in air travel has meant that passengers incubating disease can spread infection in less than 36 h to any corner of the globe, as was so dramatically shown in 2003 when a single index case of SARS coronavirus in Hong Kong infected others staying in the same hotel. Within a week these contacts spread the disease to countries as far apart as Vietnam, Singapore and Canada. Dissemination by jet is not restricted to humans: the introduction of West Nile virus into the USA in 1999 is widely thought to be the result of an infected mosquito hitching a ride on a flight from the Middle East to New York.

Table 2

Factors accounting for the increase in dengue fever and its sequelae

Uncontrolled urbanisation leading to overcrowding and inadequate sanitation
Unprecedented population growth, especially in Asia and India
A resurgence of *Aedes aegypti* and other species of mosquito capable of supporting replication and transmission
Declining standards of public health surveillance and infrastructure in endemic regions
Ease and expansion of air travel

A cardinal factor, however, is the progressive decline in public health infrastructure and associated surveillance programmes in countries where the virus is endemic or in areas where the vector and environmental conditions have established the potential for spread. Increasing pressure on scarce resources has resulted in the abandonment of programmes designed to prevent infections from becoming established in human populations. In their place are contingency plans focusing on crisis management and emergency measures. This trend, not confined to the developing world, has become coupled with a cessation in insecticide spraying in response to environmental concerns. Thus, *A. aegypti* has returned to areas previously declared free of the vector: the lack of effective surveillance in these expanding populations together with the pressure on limited funds for preventative medicine has combined to ensure the spread of dengue virus continues unabated.

Prospects for a dengue vaccine

Although a number of candidate vaccines are in various stages of clinical evaluation, currently there are no commercially available dengue vaccines. This is despite the development of an effective vaccine has been vigorously pursued now for nearly half a century. Progress has been frustratingly slow, largely because of the need to develop a tetravalent product that is equally effective against all four serotypes: the concern is that a monovalent vaccine specific for any one serotype might predispose a recipient to severe disease if that vaccine is later exposed to a serotype other than that present in the vaccine. The emphasis, therefore, has been on the development of a tetravalent vaccine consisting of attenuated strains of all four serotypes. Given the heterogeneity in properties other than just antigenicity between the serotypes, and between genotypes within each serotype, strain selection has been fraught with difficulties.

The emphasis on developing an attenuated vaccine has been driven by a consideration of manufacturing costs and also the perceived need for a vaccine that can be delivered as a single dose, particularly if realistic immunisation protocols are to be developed. Chemical inactivation of wild type virus has received considerably less attention for these very reasons, with chemical inactivation carrying an additional risk of alterations to the structural properties of the virus to such an extent that the immunogenicity of the envelope proteins is diminished. Inactivation also introduces the chance of variable damage between the different viruses going into a tetravalent product. The product profile of a putative dengue vaccine is summarised in Table 3.

Work is also hampered by the lack of a suitable animal model capable of mimicking the course of the disease in humans, particularly the progression from acute disease to DHF and DSS. Non-human primates have been used extensively but these animals, whilst supporting virus replication, do not show any manifestations of clinical disease. Thus, their use is restricted to the measurement of a reduction in viraemia that might occur in immunised animals subsequently challenged with wild type virus. The use of non-human primates also presents increasingly difficult issues of ethics and cost, the latter in particular often inhibiting the use of animals in sufficient numbers to make meaningful and statistically valid comparisons. Mice, although susceptible, present

Table 3

Product profile for a candidate dengue virus vaccine

Contains representative viral proteins from all four dengue virus serotypes
Can grow to high yields in mammalian cells
Induces a balanced response to all four components
Can be delivered as a single dose
Induce both T and B cell responses
Stimulate immunological memory (>10 years)
Does not grow in mosquitoes
Induces a low viraemia in recipients
Components are phenotypically stable and do not revert to wild type

considerable limitations. Dengue is one of the least neurotropic for mice among the flaviviruses. Nevertheless, there have been some advances using mice deficient in interferon and also with mice transplanted with human hepatocellular carcinoma cells: these animals when injected with dengue virus mimic at least some of the features of the clinical disease seen in humans (Johnson and Roehrig, 1999; An et al., 1999).

Passage in cell culture is the traditional method for attenuating virus. However, dengue virus generally produces only low titres in mammalian cells. This is a major obstacle, unless large-scale tissue culture reactors are available. These systems are expensive to maintain, however, and are often plagued by contamination as well as consuming large quantities of tissue culture media. Notwithstanding these problems, the use of modern bulk cell culture techniques means that large quantities of other flaviviruses such as Japanese encephalitis virus can now be grown to titres in excess of 10^{12} pfu/ml (quoted in Pugachev et al., 2003).

Many attempts to produce attenuated virus in cell culture have largely proved disappointing: the virus either remains too reactogenic for human use or becomes over-attenuated and as a consequence fails to induce an immune response consistently in all recipients (Kanesa-Thasan, 1998). Early experience with this work showed the importance of carefully selecting vaccine candidate strains by comparing immunogenicity with passage level. These efforts would have been helped by more information as to what constitutes suitable markers of attenuation. Nucleotide changes in the $5'$ and $3'$ NTR regions or amino acid changes in NS1 and NS3 leading to the appearance of small plaque variants, reduced replication in mosquitoes, as such are all potentially useful *in vitro* correlates of the extent to which virulence has been modified by cell passage.

The most promising attenuated vaccine candidates have been developed at Mahidol University in Bangkok. Candidate viruses representing each serotype were prepared by sequential passage, first in primary dog kidney cells, then in either primary African green monkey kidney cells or in foetal rhesus lung cells (Rothman et al., 2001). The complexity of these studies is illustrated by the titre of each vaccine candidate (equating to a 50% infectious dose) recovered from the blood of human volunteers. These titres were 10^4, 5, 3500 and 150 pfu for serotypes 1–4, respectively, i.e. representing a four $\log_{10}$ difference in response against the four serotypes. This makes for considerable problems in formulating a tetravalent vaccine. Phase I trials of a tetravalent vaccine have been conducted using these candidates using approximately $3-4 \log_{10}$ of virus per inoculum. There were no serious adverse events associated with this vaccine, although recipients complained of headaches, a mild fever ($\sim 38°C$) and a macropapular rash that was sometimes puritic. There was evidence of a viraemia in all volunteers from 5 to 12 days after injection (Kanesa-Thasan et al., 2001). The highest anti-dengue virus antibody titres were present against dengue 3, and only dengue 3 was recovered consistently from viraemic blood samples. Despite the equivalence of dose, the data suggested that either the dengue 3 virus component was not sufficiently attenuated or that competitive interference occurred. Slightly more encouraging was the finding of proliferative and cytotoxic T-lymphocyte responses against all the serotypes except dengue 4 (Rothman et al., 2001). These results show just how much of an uphill task the process of developing a tetravalent vaccine represents.

Other more traditional approaches to developing live attenuated vaccines include exposure of wild type isolates to mutagenic chemicals followed by a process of selecting those mutated viruses with evidence of reduced virulence. This approach has not received nearly as much attention for developing a dengue vaccine, however. Blaney et al. (2001) followed this route to modify a dengue 4 candidate previously shown to give rise to fever and a rash in volunteers despite a deletion in the $3'$ NTR. A number of temperature-sensitive mutants were recovered after exposure to the mutagen 5-fluorouracil: these all showed a reduced ability to grow in mice brains.

An alternative approach exploits the observation made by Bray and Lai (1991) that the structural genes of one dengue virus serotype can be exchanged for the homologous genes of another. These investigators successfully generated chimeras by taking a dengue 4 clone and replacing all of the structural genes (C, prM and E) with those of dengue 1, dengue 2 or dengue 3. The chimeras grew well in monkey kidney cells and mosquito C6-36 cells and induced high titres of neutralising antibodies in monkeys (Table 4). This work was taken further by attenuating the dengue 4 template by introducing non-lethal mutations at the $5'$ and $3'$ NTRs. This technology has been extended still further by replacing the dengue 4 template with that of the PDK strain of dengue 2, a component of the attenuated, tetravalent vaccine described above. As yet the immunogenic potential of these chimeras has only been reported using mice (Huang et al., 2000).

Table 4

Neutralising antibody titres in rhesus monkeys injected with one or two doses of chimeric yellow fever/dengue virus (from Guirakhoo et al., 2002)

Virus chimera	Geometric mean titre (GMT)		
	First dose	Second dose	P value
Yellow fever/DEN1	640	1810	0.12
Yellow fever/DEN2	1437	1613	0.80
Yellow fever/DEN3	640	1016	0.26
Yellow fever/DEN4	3225	5120	0.01

Given the demonstration of chimera formation between serotypes of dengue, it is not surprising that chimera vaccines have been attempted using the yellow fever vaccine strain 17D. This methodology is being commercialised by Acambis Inc.[4] as ChimeraVax™. Experience with Japanese encephalitis virus—also a mosquito-borne flavivirus—showed that the replacement of genes between different flaviviruses was restricted to the envelope proteins prM and E. The Japanese encephalitis (JE) chimera was significantly less lethal for suckling mice compared to the 17D virus. Important from the point of its potential use in humans, the 17D-JE chimera did not replicate in either *Aedes* or *Culex* mosquitoes. The development of these new immunogens is described further by Pugachev et al. (2003).

Viable yellow fever 17D/dengue chimeras have been produced for all of the dengue serotypes (Guirakhoo et al., 2001). These have been constructed using clones expressing the prM and E proteins of wild type isolates from different localities. These chimeras are significantly less virulent for mice compared to the 17D virus. All grew to a high titre in Vero cells, a significant advantage compared to wild type dengue isolates. Experiments in rhesus monkeys have shown only low viraemias but the presence of specific B cell responses. Encouragingly the induced neutralising antibodies were sufficient to protect the animals against challenge with wild type virus. Although these data are encouraging, the adjustment of the dose for each individual component is as much of a problem as when a tetravalent vaccine was used composed of attenuated virus strains. However, a uniform antibody response to all four serotypes could be achieved by giving a second dose 60 days after the first (Guirakhoo et al., 2002). Importantly, pre-existing antibodies to 17D virus did not affect the titre of anti-dengue virus antibodies generated by these chimeras (Table 5). At present, the ChimeraVax™ dengue 2 vaccine is the subject of phase II clinical trials (Pugachev et al., 2003).

As has been the case with many high priority vaccine development programmes, there has been intensive effort directed towards evaluating alternative approaches that avoids the need to produce large quantities of whole virus. These include sub-unit vaccines using expressed proteins from mammalian cells, insect cells or bacteria, and DNA immunogens incorporating the relevant dengue genes and recombinant vectors expressing dengue envelope genes.

Much of this effort is summarised by Kinney and Huang (2001). The key questions are, first, is one protein sufficient for the induction of protective immunity, and second, what role, if any, is played by protein conformation. Most workers agree that the envelope protein (E) is of primary importance for inducing a protective antibody response but there is a body of evidence suggesting other proteins may also be required, such as prM/M, NS1 and NS3. Certainly T cell responses can be measured against many, if not all, NS proteins in patients with flavivirus infections. It is worth remembering that the detection of antibody to the NS3 protein of hepatitis C virus gave the first clue as to the presence of this virus in cases hitherto grouped as non-A, non-B hepatitis. Recombinant hepatitis C vaccines based upon the E1 and E2 proteins have been rapidly worked up and tested as vaccine candidates. Attempts to produce a hepatitis C vaccine

---

[4] http://www.acambis.com.

have shown, however, that protein conformation is vitally important if the correct B cell specificity is to be retained and presented to the immune system.

Good responses to the E protein of dengue 4 have been obtained using recombinant vaccinia virus, even though the C-terminal part of the E protein was deleted during the cloning process (Men et al., 1991). However, lower levels of protection have been seen using similar recombinants containing the truncated E protein of Japanese encephalitis virus. It is now known that one of the major roles of prM is to ensure the correct folding of E (Lorenz et al., 2002): probably for this reason the expression of subviral particles containing both prM and E also induces good titres of neutralising antibodies (Fonseca et al., 1994).

New advances in molecular virology have led to the generation of infectious clones. Attenuation of the potential virulence of such clones has focused on modifications to both the 5′ and 3′ NTR.[5] For example, Men et al. (1996) took an infectious clone of dengue 4 and deleted sequences in the 3′ NTR. These clones produced smaller plaques in cell culture and a lower viraemia in monkeys. This initial finding was sufficient to encourage a small human trial in 20 volunteers using one clone with the 30 nucleotides deleted spanning bases 172–143 reading from the 3′ end. A low titre viraemia was confirmed in 14, with neutralising antibodies found in all cases (Durbin et al., 2001). This and other clones with 3′ NTR modifications do not grow well in mosquitoes and mosquito cell cultures. Care will have to be taken using single point mutations to generate this type of attenuated vaccine clone, however, as there is evidence of phenotypic reversion to wild type over prolonged periods of growth in C6-36 cells (Markoff et al., 2002).

Kyasanur Forest disease

Kyasanur Forest disease was first isolated in 1957 from a dead monkey found in Mysore (now Karnataka) in India, and is hence known locally as monkey fever. This followed a series of unexplained deaths among monkeys living in the Kyasanur Forest. In contrast to Omsk haemorrhagic fever (see below), there are a steady number of cases reported each year, predominantly among villagers living at the forest margins. A number of laboratory infections have also been reported.

Epidemiology

Kyasanur Forest disease virus is transmitted by the bite of the tick *Haemaphysalis spinigera*, a tick often found at the forest margins. Rodents, bats and shrews as well as monkeys are also susceptible to the virus. This disease has most likely emerged as a consequence of extensive forest clearing to make way for cattle grazing. This in turn has led to a rise in tick populations and thus an increase in risk of human exposure. Forest rodents are the most likely host reservoirs, monkeys and man serving as only coincidental hosts, with infected primates serving to amplify outbreaks.

---

[5] NTR: Non-translated regions at the end of a viral genome.

Clinical features

A sudden fever rising rapidly to 40°C is accompanied by myalgia and headache, these early symptoms closely resembling those of dengue fever. In contrast to dengue fever, however, muscle pain is localised in the upper thorax and neck. A helpful early sign is the appearance of vesicular lesions on the upper palate. A lymphadenopathy is usually present. Haemorrhagic disease appears from day 3, consisting of gastrointestinal bleeding accompanied by bleeding of the gums and nose. Although there is a thrombocytopenia, there are neither indications of major disruption to the haematopoietic system nor signs of capillary damage. The occurrence of laboratory-acquired infections has allowed a more detailed study of the disease profile: these show a stronger involvement of the CNS than is evident from clinical cases, with signs of coarse tremors, abnormal reflexes and mental disturbances. Mortality is between 3 and 5%. It has been noted that naturally acquired infections occur predominantly among residents of villages with minimal or no infrastructure. These people have as a consequence a high parasitic burden and this in turn leads to elevated levels of interferon and IgE. Some workers have gone as far as suggesting that these immunological markers may play a role in determining the course of the clinical disease.

Diagnosis

As is the case with many flavivirus infections, direct virus isolation is possible from blood samples using either suckling mice or cell cultures. Antibodies can be detected using ELISA or other standard serological methods, including plaque reduction neutralisation.

Control

A formalin-inactivated vaccine has been prepared locally and preliminary clinical trials has shown good protection (Dandawate et al., 1994). This vaccine is now being produced in Bangalore, India, for local use.

Alkhurma virus

In 1995, a new flavivirus was recovered from patients with severe haemorrhagic disease in Saudi Arabia (Zaki, 1997). Of the six cases identified initially, four were proved fatal. All were butchers and it is probable that the infections were acquired as a result of handling infected sheep or coming into contact with ticks feeding on infected animals. All patients showed signs of fever, headache, generalised muscle pain, nausea and arthralgia. There was a marked thrombocytopenia and biochemical evidence of both liver and renal damage. A further four cases were identified serologically following the development of a test for IgM antibodies.

Charrel et al. (2001a,b) have sequenced the genome of Alkhurma virus and shown that it is closely related to Kyasanur Forest disease virus. It remains to be determined as to the nature of the common ancestor of these two agents and to how Alkhurma virus has emerged in a region some 2000 km away from the endemic region of Kyasanur Forest disease.

Omsk haemorrhagic fever

The endemic area is thought restricted to the Omsk and Novosibirsk-Oblast regions of Siberia, a landscape essentially of forest and steppe. Almost all the cases described in the literature occurred between 1945 and 1958, with a peak between 1945 and 1949. Sporadic outbreaks continue to occur, the most recent in 1991. Laboratory infections have also been reported, again indicating that this virus can be readily transmitted to humans.

Omsk haemorrhagic fever is transmitted by the ticks *Dermocentor reticulates* and *D. marginatus*. The virus can persist in ticks throughout the winter period, although there is no evidence of transovarial transmission. Interestingly, this virus cannot readily be distinguished from tick-borne encephalitis by use of hyperimmune antibodies: despite this close serological relationship, Omsk haemorrhagic fever causes severe disturbance to the haematological system whereas tick-borne encephalitis virus does not. The reason for this difference is not known, but lies at the heart of understanding why closely related viruses—at least on virological and serological grounds—can cause very different clinical diseases. The virus of Omsk haemorrhagic fever is maintained in nature by muskrats (*Ondatra zibethica*) and water voles (*Arvicola terrestris*). The muskrat is a recent introduction into this region and is highly susceptible to the virus. The infection rapidly progresses in this species to a fulminant, haemorrhagic disease that is invariably fatal. It is the hunters of the muskrat in Western Siberia and their close family members that are most at risk, with infected muskrats shedding large quantities of virus in urine and faeces. Hunters become exposed when skinning infected animals. Family members of these hunters account for approximately a quarter of human cases reported so far, indicating that human-to-human transmission can readily occur between close contacts.

Clinical features

The first signs of human infection are the sudden onset of fever accompanied by myalgia and headache. Haemorrhagic manifestations quickly follow with epistaxis and gastrointestinal bleeding. A bronchial pneumonia is frequently present, and only occasionally is there an indication of CNS involvement (Pavri, 1989). The case fatality rate is less than 3%. Diagnosis is by detection of specific antibodies using serology and virus isolation from a blood sample.

Recently the complete sequence of the Bogoluvoska strain has been reported (Lin et al., 2003). Phylogenetic analysis revealed a close relationship with other viruses of the tick-borne complex in the family Flaviviridae, but sufficiently distinct as to form a separate clade, a conclusion compatible with Omsk haemorrhagic fever virus only having minimal neurotropism. The glycoprotein (E) of Omsk haemorrhagic fever virus is also distinct from that of Kyasanur Forest disease and Alkhurma viruses, two other tick-

Table 5

Flaviviruses—key questions

Why yellow fever does not occur in parts of the world where vectors exist with the potential for disease transmission?

What is the mechanism by which yellow fever vaccines confer protection?

How can dengue vaccines be developed against all four serotypes whilst minimising the risk of disease enhancement by sequential exposure to different serotypes?

What are the underlying pathological mechanisms giving rise to dengue haemorrhagic fever and shock syndrome?

What is the risk posed to human health by viruses such as Kyasanur Forest disease outside of their present endemic areas?

---

transmitted flaviviruses with the capacity to induce haemorrhagic disease. A detailed comparison with these two and other neurotropic flaviviruses suggested only three amino acid changes correlated with the divergence in biological properties of these viruses. One of these changes, at residue 76, is close to the presumptive membrane fusion domain, the remaining two within the stem-anchor region of the protein. Further differences were noted outside of the single open reading frame, in particular the 5' NTR secondary structure of the Omsk haemorrhagic fever viral genome is likely very different, a possible reflection on the unique virus–vector relationship of the virus with ticks of the *Dermocentor* genus. Although speculative, it is clear that Omsk haemorrhagic fever virus has adapted to a particular vector and ecological niche quite separate from those of other tick-borne flaviviruses co-circulating in Siberia.

Control

Prevention of disease can be accomplished readily by avoidance of ticks and taking care when handling dead muskrats. No vaccine is available, although there is an opinion that the serological relationship between Omsk haemorrhagic fever and tick-borne encephalitis virus is sufficiently close that the administration of tick-borne encephalitis vaccines to those at risk is beneficial. Although not indicated for Omsk haemorrhagic fever, vaccines against tick-borne encephalitis virus were used in Siberia to control the 1991 outbreak under a special directive of the regional authorities.

Summary

The spectrum of diseases caused by flaviviruses range from the encephalitic to the viscerotropic in terms of pathology. It is the latter that have the propensity to various haemorrhagic manifestations. Despite the availability of vaccines against yellow fever represents one of the major achievements of modern medicine, this very achievement is under threat as major yellow fever outbreaks can rapidly lead to vaccine shortages and attempts to curb childhood yellow fever by introducing the vaccine into childhood immunisation programmes has faltered in recent years. Coupled with the resurgence of

A. aegypti in major conurbations—especially in the Americas—the scene is set for outbreaks on a scale not seen for over a century and there is a very real risk that these may not be fully contained if vaccine is in short supply. The threat posed to public health by dengue virus is considerable, this virus having gone a major expansion in endemicity in the last 50 years to affect over 50 countries. There has been a corresponding escalation in the number of cases of DHF and shock syndrome, especially among younger patients. Despite dengue virus now being the most widespread of all the viral haemorrhagic fevers, licensed vaccines are still not in sight, largely due to the hurdle of developing a vaccine capable of inducing protection equally against all four serotypes. Although Omsk haemorrhagic fever and Kyasanur Forest disease viruses pose problems in very restricted geographical regions, there are signs that these agents may represent the vanguard of other agents still to be discovered. The emergence of Alkhurma virus closely related to Kyasanur Forest disease virus is a worry, having been isolated in Saudi Arabia some 2000 km from the endemic zone of Kyasanur Forest disease virus. Ease of transport and further changes to the environment will only escalate the risk that flaviviruses pose to human health on a global scale. Although the short-term prospects for specific treatment with antiviral is bleak, the intensive efforts to develop new therapies for chronic hepatitis C almost certainly will generate in the longer term compounds that may prove beneficial for the treatment of a spectrum of flavivirus infections, in the same way that hepatitis B therapy has benefited enormously from the discovery of antivirals against HIV.

Arenaviruses

The arenaviruses are a family of enveloped, single-stranded RNA viruses. Few cause severe haemorrhagic diseases in man, notably Lassa fever in Africa, and Argentine haemorrhagic fever in South America. More recently, several new arenaviruses have been described from South America and the United States, three of which are associated with severe human diseases. In common with lymphocytic choriomeningitis virus (LCM), the natural reservoir of these infections is limited to a few rodent species (Howard, 1986).

Although the first isolates obtained from South America in the 1960s and 1970s were erroneously designated as newly defined arboviruses, there is no evidence to implicate arthropod transmission for any arenavirus. However, similar methods of isolation and the necessity of trapping small animals have meant historically that the majority of arenaviruses have been isolated by workers in the arbovirus field. A good example of this is Guanarito virus that emerged during investigation of a dengue virus outbreak in Venezuela (Salas et al., 1991). The discovery of Sin Nombre Virus as a cause of Hantavirus Pulmonary Syndrome has led to a resurgence of interest in the link between zoonoses and persistent virus infections of rodents (see Bunyaviruses for a description of the hantaviruses). The Four Corners outbreak of Hantavirus Pulmonary Syndrome in 1993 served to heighten awareness that fevers of hitherto unknown origin might equally be the result of infection with agents normally maintained in rodent reservoirs. This is particularly so in Argentina where virologists and clinicians specialising in Argentine Haemorrhagic Fever have been in the vanguard of national efforts linking respiratory disease with the discovery of new hantaviruses co-existing with arenaviruses in the same rodent populations. This vigilance has brought rewards in the rapid linking of severe respiratory disease with Whitewater Arroyo virus in the south-western United States.

With the current concern about so-called "emerging viruses", the arenaviruses are an excellent illustration as to how environmental changes may result in an altered balance between man and natural animal hosts, leading to unexpected diseases which can severely challenge local and national public health resources. There is a wide spectrum of pathological processes associated with these viruses giving useful insights into other zoonotic infections. Notably LCM has been used as a model of persistent virus infection for over half a century. Its study has revealed a number of cardinal concepts to our present understanding of interactions between a virus and the immune system, particularly the phenomenon of MHC restriction associated with cytotoxic T lymphocyte killing of virus-infected cells, and the role of such responses in immunologically mediated disease processes. Peter Doherty and Rolf Zinkernagel were jointly awarded the 1996 Nobel

Prize in Physiology or Medicine[1] for elucidating what has become a fundamental tenet in our understanding of how the cellular immune system eliminates cells harbouring pathogens or displaying other manifestations of an underlying disease process. At the other end of the spectrum of aenavirus pathology, all the evidence is that the morbidity of Lassa fever and South American haemorrhagic fevers due to arenavirus infection results from the direct cytopathic action of these agents, in sharp contrast to the immunopathological basis of "classic" lymphocytic choriomeningitis disease seen in adult mice infected with LCM virus.

For a general overview of the arenaviruses, see the two volume monograph edited by Michael Oldstone (Oldstone, 2002a,b). A comprehensive overview of the arenaviruses causing human disease can be found on http://www.cdc.gov/ncidad/dvrd/spb and http://www.who.int/health-topics/index.

Properties of the virus

Nomenclature and natural history

The morphological, physicochemical and serological properties of the arenaviruses were first summarised by Pfau (1974). The 23[2] current members of the family currently are listed in Table 1. The various strains and isolates of LCM are now considered to be a genus within the family Arenaviridae. A close serological relationship exists between LCM, Lassa virus and other arenaviruses from Africa. For this reason, they are loosely referred to as the "Old World" arenavirus, in contrast to those from the Americas, although LCM virus can be found worldwide except in Australia. The "New World" arenaviruses show varying degrees of serological relationships with Tacaribe virus, first isolated in Trinidad. For this reason, viruses from the Americas are frequently regarded as members of the Tacaribe complex.

The Arenaviridae take their name from the sand-sprinkled appearance when viewed in the electron microscope (Latin: *arena* = sand). With the exception of LCM, all are referred to by names that reflect the geographical area in which they were isolated (Fig. 1). Various strain designations are also commonly used, in particular for LCM and arenaviruses isolated from man. Multiple isolations of non-pathogenic viruses that infect New World rodents are made less frequently, with the exception of Pichinde virus where a large number of field isolates from Colombia have been collected and characterised. However, the recent resurgence of interest in these viruses has uncovered a number of new arenaviruses that have tentatively been described as additional members of the Arenaviridae. Several of these may be new variants of existing family members.

All but one of the 23 members of the Arenaviridae so far described have rodents as their natural reservoir hosts. Although rodents are divided into over 30 families distributed worldwide, arenaviruses are predominantly found within two major families: Muridae (mice and rats) and Cricetidae (voles, lemmings, gerbils). The nature of

[1] For citation and further details see http://www.nobel.se/medicine/laureates/1996/press.html.

[2] At the time of writing (September 2003) a further putative arenavirus has been recorded (Rio Carcarana virus).

Table 1

The arenaviruses: hosts and geographical distribution

Virus	Natural Host	Human disease	Distribution
(World Wide)			
Lymphocytic	*Mus musculus,*	Aseptic meningitis	Europe, N. and S. America
Choriomeningitis	*Mus domesticus*		
Old World			
Ippy	*Arvicanthus* spp.	Not recorded	Central African Republic
Lassa	*Mastomys natalensis*	Lassa fever	West Africa
Mobala	*Praomys jacksoni*	Infection possible	Central African Republic
Mopeia	*Mastomys natalensis*	Infection possible	Mozambique, Zimbabwe
New World			
Allpahuayo	*Oecomys* spp.	Not recorded	Peru
Amapari	*Oryzomys gaedi,*	Not recorded	Brazil
	Neocomys guianae		
Bear Canyon	*Peromyscus californicus*	Infection possible	USA
Cupixi	*Oryzomys capito*	Not recorded	Brazil
Flexal	*Neocomys* spp.	Not recorded	Brazil
Guanarito	*Sigmodon alstoni,*	Venezuelan haemorrhagic	Venezuela
	Zygodontomys brevicuda	fever	
Junín	*Calomys musculimus, C.,*	Argentine haemorrhagic	Argentina
	Laucha Akadon azarae	fever	
Latino	*Calomys callosus*	Not recorded	Bolivia
Machupo	*Calomys callosus*	Bolivian haemorrhagic	Bolivia
		fever	
Pampa	*Bolomys sp.*	Not recorded	Argentina
Paraná	*Oryzomys buccinatus*	Not recorded	Paraguay
Pichinde	*Oryzomys albigularis*	Not recorded	Columbia
Pirital	*Sigmodon alstoni*	Not recorded	Venezuela
Oliveros	*Bolomys obscurus*	Not recorded	Argentina
Sabiá	Unknown	Brazilian haemorrhagic	Brazil
		fever	
Tacaribe	*Artibeus literatus (bat)*	Infection possible	Trinidad
Tamiami	*Sigmodon hispidus*	Not recorded	Florida, USA
Whitewater Arroyo	*Neotoma albigula*	Not recorded	New Mexico, USA

the original reservoir for LCM virus remains obscure, but it appears to be mainly in species of the Muridae which evolved in the Old World and subsequently spread to most parts of the globe. Interestingly, there is a wide range of tropism and virulence among those strains of LCM virus originally isolated from laboratory mouse colonies.

The natural reservoirs of Lassa virus and the remaining Old World arenaviruses are members of the genus Mastomys. This is also a member of the Muridae and, in common with the host of LCM virus, frequents human dwellings and food stores. In contrast, nearly all arenaviruses isolated from the South American continent are associated with cricetid rodents whose members frequent open grasslands and forest. The exception is Tacaribe virus, which was originally isolated from the fruit bat, *Artibeus literatus*.

56

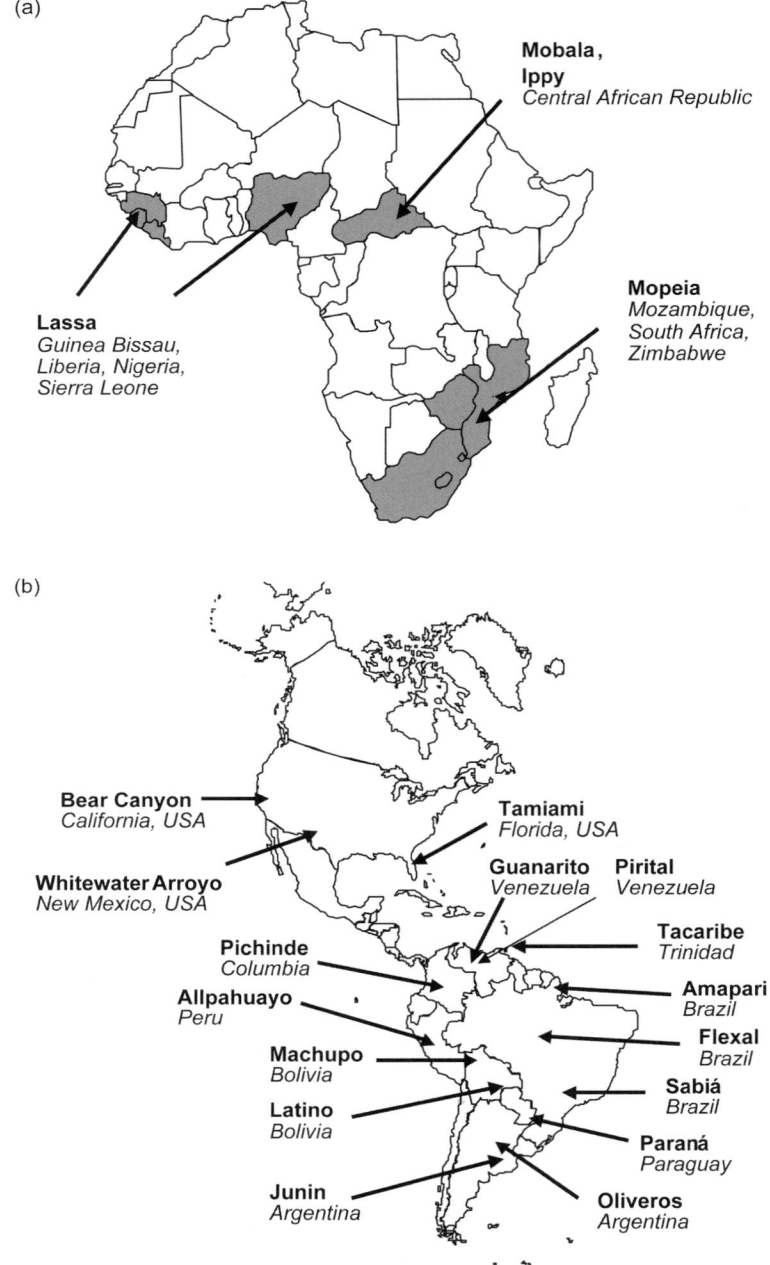

Fig. 1 Geographical distribution of Old World (a) and New World (b) arenaviruses. Lymphocytic choriomengitis virus (LCM) can be found on all continents except Australasia.

Ultrastructure of arenaviruses and infected cells

Negative-staining electron microscopy of extracellular virus shows pleomorphic particles ranging in diameter from 80 to 150 nm (Fig. 2). The virus envelope is formed from the plasma membrane of infected cells. A significant thickening of both bilayers of the membrane together with an increase in the width of the electron-translucent intermediate layer is characteristic of arenavirus maturation. Little is known about the internal structure of the arenavirus particle, although thin sections of mature and budding viruses clearly show the ordered, and often circular, arrangements of host ribosomes that are typical of this virus group. This appearance confers the "sandy" appearance from which the name of these viruses is derived. Distinct well-dispersed filaments 5–10 nm in diameter are released from detergent-treated virus. Two predominant size classes are present, with average lengths of 649 and 1300 nm, respectively; these lengths do not show a close relationship with the two virus-specific L and S RNA species. Each is circular and beaded in appearance. Convoluted filamentous strands up to 15 nm in diameter can be seen in preparations of spontaneously disrupted Pichinde virus.

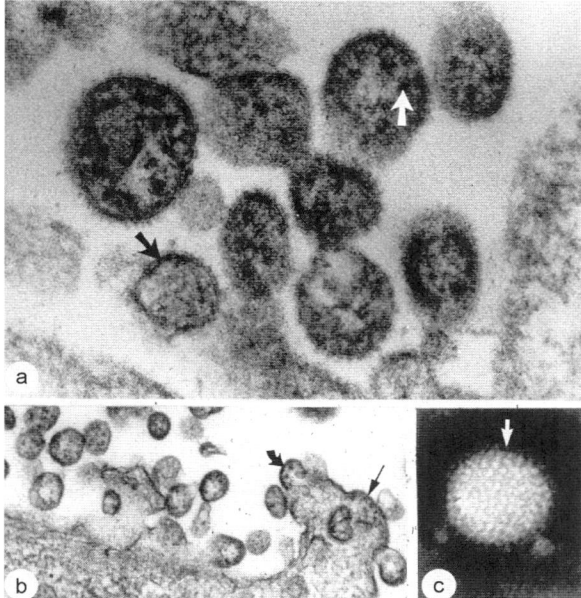

Fig. 2 Electron microscopy of arenaviruses. (a) Thin section of Lassa fever virus particles showing the internal ribosomes (white arrow) which give rise to the unique "sandy" appearance of arenaviruses, (b) Thin section of Lassa fever particles budding from an infected Vero cell. The arrows show the thickened plasma membrane at the site of virus maturation that is a feature of cells infected with arenaviruses. (c) Negatively stained Lassa fever virus particles approximately 120 nm in diameter showing the outer envelope covered with surface glycoproteins (micrographs by kind permission of Dr D.S. Ellis).

These appear to represent globular condensations which arise from an association between neighbouring turns of the underlying helix. The basic configuration of the filaments shows a linear array of globular units up to 5 nm in diameter, probably representing single molecules of the viral polypeptide. These filaments progressively fold through a number of intermediate helical structures to produce the stable 15 nm diameter forms (Young, 1987).

Arenaviruses replicate in experimental animals in the absence of any gross pathological effect. However, cellular necrosis may accompany virus production, not unlike that seen in virus-infected cell cultures. The variable pathological changes associated with arenavirus infections are further complicated by the occasional appearance of particles in tissue sections that react strongly with fluorescein-conjugated antisera. Granular fluorescence with convalescent serum in the perinuclear region of acutely infected Vero cells is often seen. In addition, intracytoplasmic inclusion bodies are a prominent feature in virus-infected cells both *in vitro* and *in vivo*. These usually appear early in the replication cycle and consist largely of single ribosomes which later become condensed in an electron-dense matrix, sometimes together with fine filaments (Murphy and Whitfield, 1975).

Chemical composition

Proteins

All arenaviruses contain a major nucleocapsid-associated protein of molecular weight 60–68,000 with two glycoproteins in the outer viral envelope. These envelope glycoproteins are not primary gene products but arise by proteolytic cleavage of a larger, 75,000 molecular weight glycoprotein precursor polypeptide (GPC). Maturation and release of virus do not seem to be markedly inhibited in the presence of tunicamycin, an inhibitor of glycosylation, but glycoprotein processing is essential for infectivity.

The major glycoprotein species (GP2) in the molecular weight range of 34–42,000 represents the C-terminal cleavage product of the GPC envelope glycoprotein precursor. The first 59 amino acids at the N-terminus of GPC act as a signal sequence, containing two distinct hydrophobic domains that could function during glycoprotein transport and virus assembly. GP1 is cleaved from the N-terminus at a unique cleavage site that is conserved among all arenaviruses except Tacaribe. GP1 assembles into tetramers linked by disulphide bonds. GP2 is also thought to form tetrameric structures proximal to GP1 in the glycoprotein peplomer, penetrating the viral membrane to form electrovalent bonds with the underlying N-RNA nucleocapsid complexes. Recent studies suggest interactions with the Z protein may also mediate peplomer formation during virus maturation.

A major antigenic site recognised by antibodies has been located between amino acids 390 and 405, and cross-reactive monoclonal antibodies bind epitopes in this region. The corresponding N-terminal product of GPC cleavage (GP1) is probably highly glycosylated with at least four antigenic domains. Neutralising monoclonal antibodies to LCM virus map to two of these regions and there is less sequence homology between the GP1 than between the GP2 molecules of different arenaviruses. Polyclonal neutralising antibody appears to react predominantly with conformation-dependent structures within one of these domains.

The internal nucleocapsid-associated (N) protein accounts for over 70% of the proteins present in purified virus and infected cells, and remains bound to the virus genome after solubilisation of the virus to form structures resembling the string of beads seen by electron microscopy. Cleavage products of the N protein are a consistent feature of both the virus and virus-infected cells. Cleavage is not noticeable in Vero cells; yields of arenaviruses are lower in these cells, perhaps due to reduced availability of N for packaging. N protein accumulates in the cytoplasm, with a fragment of the N protein often seen in the nuclei, the exact function of which is not clear. Molecular cloning studies have shown a surprisingly high degree of homology between the 558 and 570 amino acid N proteins of Old and New World arenaviruses with structural motifs and RNA-binding domains particularly conserved. This would account for the serological cross-reactions seen using certain monoclonal antibodies raised against such epidemiologically distinct viruses and may indicate precise functional roles in virus replication for certain domains of the N polypeptide.

A minor component with a molecular weight in excess of 150,000 is often observed in infected cells and is found with purified nucleocapsids. This L protein is coded by the larger RNA genome segment as shown by the study of reassortment viruses and represents the virus-specific RNA polymerase (Fuller-Pace and Southern, 1989; Lukashevich et al., 1997). Amino acid sequences common to all RNA-dependent RNA polymerases are present along the open reading frame coding for the L protein, which suggest the conservation of certain functional domains. An additional two sequences are shared with the RNA polymerases of bunyaviruses.

The Z gene product is a highly conserved, 77 amino acid polypeptide, with a central finger, or RING domain. This binds two zinc atoms in a cross-hatch arrangement (Borden et al., 1998). It is found within extracellular virus particles (Salvato et al., 1992). There is no apparent counterpart with proteins expressed by other RNA viruses. The Z protein was first considered as playing a role in controlling the replication and expression of the genome owing to its zinc-binding properties, but as will be discussed below it is now apparent that Z protein fulfils a variety of functions as a result of interactions with cellular proteins. The Z protein may also modulate the interferon response to infection *in vivo* by binding to the nuclear oncoprotein PML (Djavani et al., 2001).

Nucleic acid

The genome of arenaviruses consists of two single-stranded RNA segments of different sizes, designated L and S, with S RNA being more abundant. Analysis of RNA is complicated by the presence of ribosomal 18S and 28S RNA, although these cellular RNA species are not essential for virus replication. The total ribosomal RNA content may in turn be influenced by the varying proportions of infectious to non-infectious particles present in virus stocks, particularly if cells are infected at a multiplicity above 0.1. In addition there are small quantities of both cell and viral low molecular weight RNA.

One of these species, mRNA coding for the viral Z protein, may have a role in the initial stages of infection. There is no obvious role for these host RNA molecules in either replication or the establishment of persistent infections (see Section "Replication").

Extracted virion RNA is not infectious and the detection of a viral RNA polymerase led to the belief that arenaviruses adopt a negative-strand coding strategy with respect to viral protein synthesis. However, the actual coding strategy from the L and S RNA strands is not entirely in accord with all negative-strand RNA viruses as some genetic information can only be expressed by a genomic sense mRNA. This "ambisense" strategy is also a characteristic of some bunyavirus genomes (see Bunyaviruses). Such a coding strategy allows for the independent regulation of arenavirus envelope and nucleocapsid proteins (Fig. 4).

All arenavirus genomes have a conserved 3'-terminus at the ends of the L and S RNA; this sequence is inversely complementary to the 5'-terminus of the same RNA strand. An almost exact complementary sequence at the 5' end of both strands means that both RNA molecules adapt panhandle structures (Salvato and Shimomaye, 1989). This is in accord with the visualisation of circular ribonucleoprotein complexes extracted from whole virus (Young and Howard, 1983).

Arenavirus definition and the role of phylogenetic analysis

Rapid and accurate sequencing of viruses has transformed the manner and speed by which new isolates are analysed, offering insights into virus evolution, epidemiology and the origin of many infectious diseases. This takes particular importance when the patterns and spread of infections need to be quickly identified during the course of epidemics. Presently, such methods can raise questions as to when new isolates truly represent new arenaviruses rather than variants occupying the same ecological niche. The problems associated with defining new arenaviruses are compounded by the difficulty of measuring neutralising antibody *in vitro* using plaque reduction methods, the test generally most appropriate for defining new viruses.

The International Committee for the Taxonomy of Viruses (ICTV), an international body charged with overseeing virus taxonomy, defines a virus species as "a polythetic class of viruses that constitutes a replicating lineage and occupies a particular ecological niche". A new arenavirus would thus be defined as one differing in two or more of the criteria listed in Table 2 (Clegg, 2002). Thus the various strains of LCM virus

Table 2

Criteria as applied to defining a new member of the family Arenaviridae, as published by the International Committee for the Taxonomy of Viruses

---

Presence in a defined geographical area
An aetiological agent (or not) of disease in humans
Significant differences in antigenic cross-reactivity, including a lack of cross-neutralisation activity where applicable
Significant amino acid difference from other species in the genus
An association with a specific host species, or a group of species

---

(Pasteur, Armstrong, WE, etc.) are all variants of the prototype LCM virus and do not constitute separate species, despite the differences in pathology seen in infected mice. In contrast, Lassa and Mopeia are quite distinct species: each has a different geographical distribution despite having the same (*Mastomys natalensis*) rodent host, react differently with monoclonal antibodies, with only Lassa virus causing a disease in humans.

Although the sequencing of PCR products gives useful quantitative comparisons between newly discovered isolates and those already characterised, caution is needed both in the choice of primer sets and the method of analysis. The evolution of a single gene may not be representative of the variation of the whole genome, especially if genes that express antigenically reactive proteins are sequenced. For this reason, there has been a tendency to focus on the nucleocapsid (N) gene. Bowen et al. (1997) analysed at least one strain of all arenaviruses known at that time using maximum parsimony to generate an unrooted phylogenetic tree (Fig. 3). The results confirmed that the distant relationship between Old World and New World arenaviruses are broadly consistent with the previously determined serological relationships using polyclonal and monoclonal antibodies.

The New World arenaviruses are divisible into three lineages: clade A contains the viruses Pichinde, Tamiami, Paraná and Flexal; clade B has the viruses Sabiá, Tacaribe, Amaparí, Guanarito and the human pathogens Machupo and Junín; and clade C

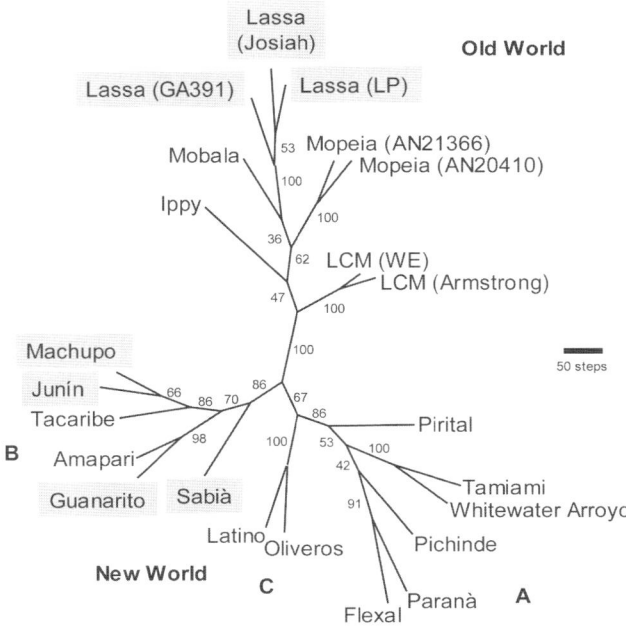

Fig. 3 Phylogenetic analysis of Old and New World arenaviruses using nucleocapsid (N) gene sequences. The New World viruses are divisible into at least three clades (From Clegg, 2002).

consists of Oliveros and Latino viruses. Interestingly, Whitewater Arroyo Virus isolated in the USA appears closely related to Tamiami, until recently the only arenavirus found in North America. However, full-length analysis of Whitewater Arroyo Virus S RNA strand has shown a quite separate ancestry for the nucleocapsid (N) and envelope (GP1, GP2) proteins, almost certainly the result of recombination between two ancestral arenaviruses (Charrel et al., 2001a,b). The N gene is clearly related to that of Pichinde and Pirital viruses, whilst its envelope glycoprotein genes resemble more those of Junín, Sabia and Tacaribe viruses. There exists less variability among the Old World members. As may be expected from their natural history, Mopeia and Mobala viruses are closely related to Lassa fever virus. The relationship revealed by phylogenetic analysis is consistent with LCM virus occupying the most ancestral position and, by and large, is confirmed by identified serological relationships and cross-protection studies in primates and guinea pigs.

Albarino and colleagues (1998) suggested that Pichinde and Oliveros viruses may be more closely related to Old World viruses when the envelope genes GP1 and GP2 are analysed in isolation. Although Clegg (2002) points out that these authors have not given sufficient weight to the greater interspecies genetic differences among the New world arenaviruses, it is intriguing that Pichinde alone is difficult to neutralise with antibody *in vitro*, a property in common with Lassa and the Old World arenaviruses.

Arenavirus evolution, rodents and human disease

Assuming that the phylogenetic trees obtained to date reflect the evolution of the whole genome, they show that the propensity of these viruses to cause severe haemorrhagic disease in humans has evolved on two distinct occasions. The South American pathogens are all confined to clade B, suggesting these viruses have acquired the capacity to infect humans as a result of a common mutational event. This phenotype must have evolved independently among the Old World viruses. Lassa fever virus has likely acquired its ability to cause serious haemorrhagic disease in humans by a quite separate evolutionary event. LCM virus can cause a quite different febrile illness, particularly if acquired from hamsters. The neurological involvement of LCM virus is an independent characteristic that almost certainly predates arenaviruses acquiring the capacity to induce haemorrhagic disease. In his book *Guns, Germs and Steel*, Jared Diamond (1997) has advocated that the human species migrated out of Africa, reaching the Americas in comparatively recent times by transversing the Bering Land Bridge. Humans advanced into South America comparatively late, around 10,000 BC. If there was no chance of arenaviruses being carried across the Atlantic and Diamond is correct, it is tempting to speculate that there is a spectrum of arenaviruses awaiting discovery in the Middle East and Asia.

Arenaviruses have adapted very precisely to their host reservoirs. Co-evolution with animal species has been demonstrated for hepesviruses and it is evident in the evolution of the genus hantavirus of the family Bunyaviridae, hantaviruses having evolved some 100 million years ago. Data is not so widely available for arenaviruses, thus making it difficult to map virus phylogeny onto that of host divergence. There is some evidence of host switching, i.e. arenaviruses crossing rodent species, adding a further complication.

In this instance the second host species acquires the virus and subsequently maintains the lineage which evolved in the original host species.

There is circumstantial evidence of co-evolution with rodent species. The increased genetic distances among New World arenaviruses is compatible with extraordinary radiation of species that occurred once Sigmontine rodents crossed the Panamanian Isthmus. This variability by far exceeds the variability seen among rodents in the Old World. Closely related South American viruses such as Junín and Machupo are found in rodent species belonging to the same genus, and clade B viruses are predominantly associated with rodents belonging to the Oryzomycini tribe. Other indications include the monophyletic relationship of Paraná, Flexal and Pichindé viruses with rodent species of the *Oryzomys* genus. The situation is less clear among the Old World arenaviruses, where considerable confusion exists as to the taxonomic relatedness between *Mastomys* and *Praomys* species within the family Murinae.

Replication

Arenaviruses replicate in a wide variety of mammalian cells, although either BHK-21 cells or monkey kidney cell lines are preferred for molecular studies (Howard, 1986). Arenaviruses can also infect a number of primary human cell lines and macrophages, including some members of the family that do not otherwise cause human infections. Most arenaviruses also grow well in mouse L cells but the simultaneous production of C-type retroviruses restricts the usefulness of such cells. The widely conserved cell protein α-dystroglycan has been identified as the cellular receptor for Old World arenaviruses, such as Lassa fever and Mobala, and those New World arenaviruses Latino and Oliveros in clade C (Cao et al., 1998). Other cell surface proteins and co-factors may also be involved, however.

At low multiplicities of infection (i.e. below 0.1) the latent period is approximately 6–8 h, after which cell-associated virus increases exponentially. The titre of extracellular virus reaches a maximum 36–48 h after infection. The passage history of any particular virus stock is probably one of the most critical factors in determining the kinetics of arenavirus replication.

Infected cells undergo only limited cytopathic changes in the cell lines commonly employed, with little or no change in the total level of host cell protein synthesis; virus yields vary in different susceptible cell types. Plaque assays are possible, but only under well-defined conditions. Cultures of persistently infected cells are readily established, with morphology and growth kinetics similar to those of uninfected cells.

The S strand codes for the nucleoprotein (N) and the envelope glycoprotein precursor (GPC) in two main open reading frames located on the same RNA molecule but with opposite polarity. The 3' half of the S RNA codes for the N protein by production of an mRNA from the S RNA strand. Although the GPC open reading fame is of positive polarity, it is not expressed until the S RNA has undergone at least a single cycle of replication, the GPC mRNA being transcribed from a template complementary in sequence to the viral genome. Thus expression of the genome is by synthesis of sub-genomic RNA from full-length templates with opposite polarities. The reading frames for the two major gene products are separated by a hairpin structure of approximately 20 paired nucleotides. This intergenic region may act as a control mechanism for genome expression by forming stable stem-loop structures that in turn regulate transcription. The S RNA of Tacaribe and Junín viruses are thought to form a second stem-loop structure.

The L RNA strand represents about 70% of the viral genome; reassortment studies with virulent and avirulent strains of LCM virus have shown that the lethality of the disease in guinea pigs is associated with the properties of the L RNA. The L protein is encoded by a large open reading frame covering 70% of the L RNA strand; it is expressed via mRNA complementary in sense to the viral genome. The mRNA for the Z protein is also expressed from the L RNA strand, probably by production of mRNA directly from the viral L strand in a manner similar to the expression of the N protein from the S strand.

The major feature of an ambisense coding strategy is that it allows for independent expression and regulation of the N and GPC genes from the S RNA segment (Fig. 4). The N protein is expressed late in acute infection and continues to be expressed in persistently infected cells in the absence of glycoprotein production. This is explained by the production of a sub-genomic mRNA from a negative polarity, virus-sense template. A control mechanism must therefore exist which determines the fate of nascent RNA of negative polarity, destined either for encapsidation or as a template for N protein-specific mRNA. In contrast, the template for glycoprotein-specific mRNA is of complementary sense to viral RNA and as such would not be required for nascent virus production. The lack of glycoprotein late in the replicative cycle or in persistently infected cells would therefore imply selective transcriptional or translational control of this gene product.

Both viral RNA and its complementary strand contain at least one intergenic region (hairpin) sequence which may provide recognition points for termination of transcription by the viral RNA polymerase. The nucleotide sequence in the hairpin region is of coding sense and may be transcribed, either as a discrete mRNA species or as a result of extended transcription of N or GPC messengers through this region. The reading frames for viral gene products transcribed from LCM and Pichinde viral genomes would fit this hypothesis. In addition, a sequence for ribosomal 18S subunit binding is present on both mRNA molecules, although its significance remains uncertain.

It is increasingly evident that the Z protein plays a role in modulating genome transcription and replication. By use of a mini-genome system, Lopez et al. (2001) showed the Z protein inhibits both transcription and replication. This interaction between Z and the polymerase (L) protein is dose-dependent and requires the RING domain. Z mediates its effect most likely by first binding and then inducing a structural change in the polymerase (Jacamo et al., 2003).

More recently, the multifunctional role of the Z protein in virus replication was revealed by the finding of Perez et al. that the Z protein effectively substituted for the late domain of the retrovirus *gag* protein. In other words, Z protein can instigate virus budding and the formation of virus-like particles in a manner similar to that of the matrix (M) protein of negative-stranded RNA viruses. This function appears mediated

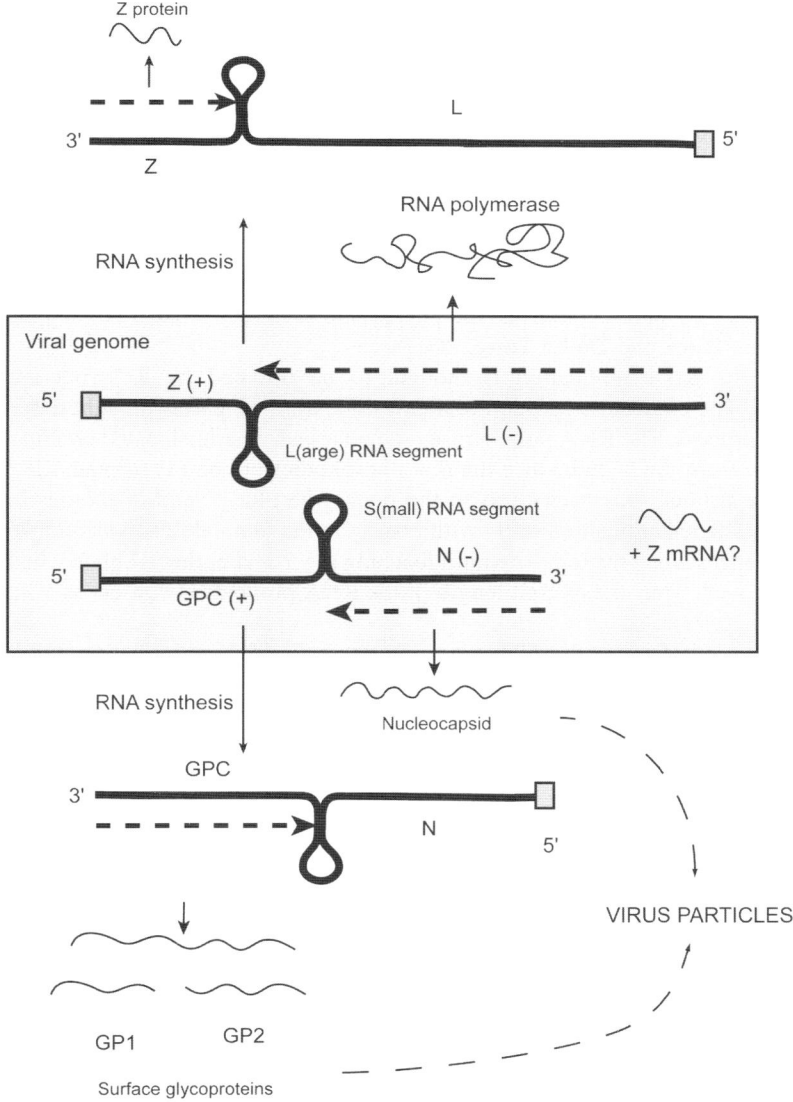

Z protein

L

3'   5'

Z

RNA polymerase

RNA synthesis

Viral genome

Z (+)

5'   3'

L (-)

L(arge) RNA segment

S(mall) RNA segment

N (-)   + Z mRNA?

5'   3'

GPC (+)

RNA synthesis

Nucleocapsid

GPC

3'

N

5'

VIRUS PARTICLES

GP1   GP2

Surface glycoproteins

Fig. 4 Arenavirus genome organisation and expression.

by two proline-rich domains separated by a short stretch of eight amino acids. Localisation of the Z protein at intracellular membranes results in recruitment of the class E vacuolar protein Tsg101, a protein also implicated in the maturation of Ebola virus (Timmins et al., 2003).

Arenavirus N protein is essential for both transcription and replication (Pinschewer, Perez, and De La Torre, 2003). Jacamo and colleagues (2003) have shown that the N protein interacts with the polymerase (L) protein via sites independent of those involved in the recognition of the Z protein, and that this interaction between N and L is an essential first step in cap-independent RNA synthesis.

The high degree of sequence conservation (17 of 19 nucleotides) at the 3' end of both L and S RNA segments is compatible with a role for these termini in promoting polymerase activity. Such terminal complementarity could thus act to nucleate the formation of new ribonucleoprotein structures by bringing together nucleoprotein (N) and nascent RNA to form a template for the viral polymerase. Work with a mini-genome of LCM virus S RNA has confirmed that this promoter is very sensitive to any nucleotide substitutions (Perez and De La Torre, 2003).

Arenavirus RNA replication is thought to be initiated by a "prime-and-align" mechanism. The enzymatic addition of a G residue to the 5' end is thought to play a key role in this process. The RNA polymerase recognises a C residue located two nucleotides downstream from the 5' end. Once the first phosphodiester bond is formed, the pppGpC dinucleotide primer slips backwards to the point when the 5' end of the nascent RNA molecule is aligned at position (-1) with respect to the template. Downstream synthesis then commences along the template until reaching the 5' end of the template when the last base is removed. Thus the overall length of the RNA products is conserved (Garcin and Kolakofsky, 1992).

Persistent infections with LCM virus are often characterised by the presence of viral RNA having either terminal deletions or extensions. Deletions would give rise to truncated genomes without the capacity to generate new virus but retain gene expression activities. Extension could repair these deletions, leading to an increase in the levels of gene expression but not sufficient to generate new infectious virus.

Epidemiology of arenavirus infections

The distribution of an arenavirus is restricted to geographical areas occupied by the corresponding rodent host. Aerosol transmission from dust and foodstuffs contaminated by rodent urine almost certainly accounts for most human infections, but there are instances where the transmission may be more complex. One example is that of Lassa fever where household cases do not necessarily match the distribution of infected *Mastomys natalensis*. However, there are many examples of laboratory-acquired arenavirus infections, confirming aerosolisation as a major risk factor. Experimental aerosol transmission to animals has been achieved for Lassa fever virus (Stephenson et al., 1984). Doses lower than 500 pfu were sufficient to induce disease in cynomolgous monkeys.

Human-to-human transmission can occur, particularly in cases of Machupo and Lassa fever virus infections. In such instances, the index case invariably was critically ill and ultimately died of the infection. Nosocomial transmission of Lassa fever virus has been especially well documented (see below). Secondary, and even tertiary, cases have been reported but these tend to occur prior to the cause of the outbreak being confirmed: the chances of further spread are reduced once the appropriate control and containment measures have been introduced. Human transmission is almost certainly related to virus load. Medical staff should always be protected by the wearing of dedicated gowns, masks and gloves, with respirators being appropriate in certain settings when the risk of nosocomial transmission is high. It is noteworthy that patients with Argentine haemorrhagic fever exhibit much lower titres of Junín virus in their blood and secretions compared to, say, patients with Lassa fever. For this reason, patients infected with Junín virus do not require the same level of strict isolation and specialist facilities.

Common to other cases of viral haemorrhagic fever, the greatest risk is parenteral transmission from contaminated needles and sharps. Autopsy is particularly hazardous (Carey et al., 1972).

Diagnosis of human arenavirus infections

The diagnosis of arenavirus infections may be made by demonstration of a fourfold rise in specific antibody titre, the presence of specific IgM antibodies, or isolation of the virus. Although arenaviruses can easily be grown in a variety of mammalian cell cultures, it must be remembered that clinical specimens from patients suspected as having a viral haemorrhagic fever should always be handled in biologically secure containment facilities. For this reason tests for antibody are more useful since inactivated viral antigens for serology can be easily prepared. For routine isolation, the E6 clone of Vero cells is the cell line of choice, although all arenaviruses grow well in primate and rodent-derived fibroblast cell lines. However, a cytopathic effect (CPE) is often difficult to see, and inoculated cultures often require examination by immunofluorescence (IF) or immunoperoxidase assay in order to detect viral antigens.

Immunofluorescence-based specific viral antibody tests are often the preferred method for the rapid diagnosis of human arenavirus infections. In the case of Lassa fever, infected cell substrates are used that have been treated by ultraviolet (UV) light, acetone, and cobalt irradiation to ensure safety. Drops of cell cultures dried onto glass slides can be prepared in a central laboratory and these preparations remain stable for many months. Most of the antigens detected within acetone-fixed infected cells represent cytoplasmic nucleocapsid protein. In the case of the New World arenaviruses, serological cross-reactions in the immunofluorescence test (e.g. with sera from patients with Bolivian (Machupo) and Argentine (Junín) haemorrhagic fevers) are found with fixed cultures. Substrates prepared from other members of the Tacaribe complex, in which Junín and Machupo viruses are categorised, also react with sera taken from these patients during the acute phase and into early convalescence. Greatest cross-reactivity is seen between the closely related Junín and Machupo antigens, closely followed by Tacaribe virus-infected cells. ELISA has been used as an alternative to immunofluorescence for early and rapid diagnosis; its use was restricted by the small amounts of antigen available for coating the solid phase but this has changed with the availability of recombinant antigens.

As a first step towards diagnosis, the use of PCR is increasingly used, provided primer sets are available that have been rigorously tested beforehand and the temperature cycling conditions are optimised. The need is often to give a first indication as to which of the various causes of viral haemorrhagic fever may be present, and thus it is often the case that PCR reactions need to be conducted in parallel using a range of primer sets specific for as many as six different agents, whether these be arenaviruses or other suspected causes, for example filoviruses. Drosten et al. (2002) have shown that this is possible, overcoming the common problems of low sensitivity and non-specific amplification often associated with such multiplex PCR tests. Most experience has been obtained for the rapid diagnosis of Junín virus (for example, see Bockstahler et al., 1992; Lozano et al., 1995). The advantages of PCR include the opportunity to obtain sequence information, of increasing relevance to the identification of new family members. Also PCR is useful for diagnosis in the early stages of disease when antibodies are yet to develop. The drawback, however, is that PCR does not discriminate between the presence of RNA fragments and infectious virus. Thus isolation of virus using cell cultures in a high-security facility should be attempted whenever possible.

Antigenic relationships

Monoclonal antibodies are used to distinguish between virus strains because they can be prepared against epitopes which go unrecognised when polyclonal antisera are used. Buchmeier et al. (1981) summarised the patterns of reactivity with a panel of monoclonal antibodies directed against laboratory strains of the homologous LCM virus, and Lassa and Mopeia viruses. Antibodies directed against the smaller, GPC envelope glycoprotein cross-reacted by immunofluorescence with all substrates examined, whereas antibodies directed against the larger GP1 glycoprotein were either strain specific or reacted with only a subset of strains, presumably by binding to previously unrecognised epitopes. The observation that certain of these broadly cross-reactive antibodies also reacted with Pichinde virus suggests that epitopes on surface envelope structures among Old World and New World arenaviruses are conserved. A similar comparison has also been undertaken with monoclonal antibodies to Lassa tested against the Mopeia and Mobala viruses from Africa. Again, various degrees of cross-reactivity were observed with reagents specific for the GP2 external glycoprotein. Mobala virus from the Central African Republic, however, appears to be distinct, as several cross-reactive monoclonal antibodies originally prepared against LCM virus failed to recognise Mobala-infected substrates. Clegg and Lloyd (1984) analysed an extensive range of different determinants common to all strains of both viruses on the internal nucleocapsid and on at least one of the two glycoproteins.

The plaque reduction neutralisation test is a highly specific method for identifying some members of the Arenaviridae, most notably those from South America. Few examples of cross-reactivity have been obtained with high-titre animal antisera raised against Junín, Tacaribe and Machupo viruses. However, the ease with which neutralising antibodies can be quantified varies greatly. Cross-reactions have not been observed between Junín and Machupo viruses in plaque reduction tests with human convalescent sera despite sharing a close antigenic relationship. A similar marked specificity of neutralisation has been demonstrated with LCM and Lassa fever viruses, although neutralising antibodies to Lassa virus can be detected only with great difficulty.

The sensitivity of the neutralisation test for LCM virus can be increased by incorporating either complement or anti-γ-globulin into the test system.

Clinical and pathological aspects

Immune response

The classic example of virus-induced immunopathological disease is LCM virus infection of adult mice (Casals, 1975) in which intracerebral inoculation causes severe disease and death. In contrast, if mice are infected before or shortly after birth they develop a non-pathogenic life long carrier state. The newborn mouse is immunologically immature and the virus does stimulate an immune response; in these circumstances the virus causes no illness. The immunologically mature mouse mounts an immune response following LCM virus infection and a fatal choriomeningitis results, but without evidence of neuronal damage (Lehmann-Grube, 1971). Immunosuppression, either by neonatal thymectomy or by use of anti-lymphocytic serum, protects adult mice against fatal LCM infection; the pathological damage thus appears to be immune-mediated.

The immune responses are best understood in acute infection of mice. Intraperitoneal injection of adults gives rise to an asymptomatic acute infection of 2–3 weeks' duration. Studies of such infections have resulted in a number of findings with implications beyond the field of arenavirus research. First, the description by Rowe (1954) of the immune-mediated pathology of acute LCM infection was the first demonstration that the pathogenicity of the viruses may not be solely related to their cytolytic effects. The observation that LCM virus-infected cells were lysed by cytotoxic T-cells led to the concept that recognition of a target cell requires the presence of both viral antigen and class I antigen of the host's major histocompatibility complex (Zinkernagel and Doherty, 1979). Secondly, the persistence of virus in mice infected shortly after birth has provided a model for both host and viral factors involved in the establishment and maintenance of chronic infection. The finding of virus antigen–antibody complexes in persistently infected animals shows that B-cell tolerance is not involved. Finally, activation of natural killer cell activity early in acute infection, which coincides with the production of interferon, has helped increase our knowledge of innate immunity against virus infection.

The direct demonstration of virus replication in lymphocytes is of substantial importance for understanding arenavirus pathogenesis, as these cells provide a continuing source of virus that enters the circulation and play a key role in the temporal and quantitative control of the immune response (Murphy and Whitfield, 1975). Viral antigen is present in the cells of the lymphatic system in mice persistently infected with LCM virus. Most of the virus in the blood of carrier mice is associated with approximately 2% of the total circulating lymphocyte population. Precursor or immature lymphocytes may support the replication in vitro of LCM virus when they are stimulated to proliferate by phytohaemagglutinin, in agreement with the general finding that arenaviruses grow best in actively dividing cells. Such clonal expansion may be triggered in vivo by viral antigen binding to appropriate lymphocyte receptors.

Arenaviruses can replicate in peritoneal and tissue macrophages. Virus can be recovered from mononuclear cells and macrophages of adult mice infected with LCM virus when these cells become activated as a result of the uptake of heterologous antigens. This does not occur in athymic mice, suggesting that infection of macrophages requires T-cell activity.

Interferon

Interferon is induced early in acute LCM virus infection of mice, and its appearance correlates with the appearance of infectious virus in the blood. There have been few studies of the levels of α-interferon in acute arenavirus infection of man. Elevated levels can be detected in the early stages of Argentine haemorrhagic fever, and these coincide with the onset of fever and backache. Although there is no correlation between the titres of interferon and circulating virus, Levis and Saavedra (1984) have suggested that at least some of the clinical signs may be directly attributable to interferon, particularly the depression of platelet and lymphocyte numbers that result from Junín virus infection of leucocytes and macrophages.

The role of natural killer cells in controlling arenavirus infection is not clear, although many are found in the blood and spleen of LCM virus infected mice as early as 1 day after infection. This response declines rapidly, however, until by the fourth day almost all the cytolytic immune activity is H-2 restricted.

Antibodies

Antibodies against the nucleocapsid can be detected by complement fixation (CF) and immunofluorescence early in the acute phase of most arenavirus infections. Infectious virus–antibody complexes can be detected 4 days after LCM virus infection of mice but there is no evidence that B-cell responses play a role in the pathology of the acute infection. Immunity to arenaviruses appears in general to be type-specific; an infection with one member of the family does not necessarily confer protective humoral or cellular immunity against arenaviruses that can be distinguished by neutralisation tests *in vitro*. However, cross-reactive antibodies may confer some degree of protection in some instances. For example, immunisation of guinea pigs with Tacaribe virus protects against subsequent challenge with the normally virulent Junín virus. These responses are clearly different from the secondary responses that may be induced as a result of antigenic similarities between the nucleocapsid proteins of the two viruses concerned.

Cellular immunity

The role of cellular immunity during acute LCM virus infection is manifested by a cytotoxic T-cell response associated with the clearing of virus; for example, CD8 + T-cells cultured and cloned *in vitro* and injected intravenously reduce the amount of virus 100-fold in the spleens of acutely infected mice. Cytotoxic T-cell responses are restricted by the need for activated T-cells to recognise both viral antigen and host cell proteins encoded by the H-2 region, a concept developed in LCM-infected mice which as referred to above has radically altered our concept of the mechanisms by which the infected host clears virus from infected tissues. The generation of specific cellular toxicity is related to the replication of the virus in target organs; inoculation with live virus appears necessary, as a primary cytotoxic T-cell response is not seen if the virus is inactivated. This has implications for the development of inactivated arenavirus vaccines should the stimulation of cellular immunity prove essential for protection as many workers believe. T-cell clones from mice infected with the Armstrong strain of LCM virus lyse a wide range of LCM virus strains. This finding demonstrates that cytotoxic responses to arenaviruses are haplotype-restricted but show a broad cross-reactivity for conserved viral determinants. Some of these determinants have been mapped to an immunodominant domain of GP2 between amino acids 278 and 286 (Whitton et al., 1988). Such T-cell clones can discriminate between cells infected with a given strain of virus containing only a single amino acid substitution in this region; this implies that mutations in this region of the genome may lead to selection of a virus variant with altered pathogenicity.

In contrast to LCM virus, the role of cellular immunity in Lassa virus infection seems to play only a minor role. The human host is clearly restricted in its ability to clear the virus and prevent virus replication in tissues, possibly because of an impaired cytotoxic T-cell response. The poor neutralising antibody response and the high degree of viraemia contrast sharply with those in patients with South American haemorrhagic fevers, in whom there is little viraemia and neutralising antibodies develop rapidly during acute infection. The prospects of immunotherapy thus seem poor and greater emphasis has, therefore, been placed on the use of antiviral agents (see below).

Persistent infection

Antibodies

Mice persistently infected with LCM virus produce antibodies to all the major structural proteins. This finding was contrary to the view previously held that viral persistence is established or maintained *in vivo* as a result of an absence of specific B-cell responses to some or all viral antigens. As viral proteins continue to be produced in the tissues of such animals, circulating antigen–antibody complexes are formed which can be detected by binding Clq. It is worth noting that, despite the existence of antibody to all LCM virus structural polypeptides, sera from persistently infected mice are negative by CF tests; this was the original basis for the belief that carrier animals do not produce a humoral response to this virus. Antibodies in the sera of such animals bind to the surface of virus-infected cells, but are unable to mediate complement-dependent cytolysis, suggesting that viral antigens at the plasma membrane may be either masked, thereby preventing further immune reactions, or removed by antigenic modulation. This notion would imply that persistently infected mice are deficient in viral antibody of the complement fixing subclass of IgG, but this has not been proven.

Cell-mediated immunity

Mice persistently infected with LCM virus should mount a normal T-cell response to unrelated immunogens, indicating a state of tolerance only to specific antigens. However, it has been difficult to distinguish T-cell suppression from an absence of virus-specific T-cell clones. Here it is pertinent to mention that persistence of LCM virus in mice infected at birth or *in utero* was one of the important observations made by Burnet and Fenner to support the concept of tolerance to "self" antigens. The time of infection is critical, as LCM virus infection induced 24 h after birth results in a cytotoxic T-cell response typical of acute disease. The failure of mice infected before this time to mount an adequate cytotoxic response is presumably related to maturation of T-cell function; it appears to be virus specific because adult carrier mice challenged with other unrelated arenaviruses mount normal cytotoxic T-cell responses. Thus the block appears to be either in recognition of infected cells, or in their expression of type-specific antigenic determinants. The relationship between the virus and the host immune response may be more complex than hitherto believed, however, as there is evidence for arenaviral RNA being transcribed into complementary DNA, presumably mediated by endogenous retroviral reverse transcriptase (Klenerman et al., 1997). This would imply that long-term persistence of viral gene sequences as retroviral elements results in continual low-level expression of viral proteins. Thus immune responsiveness is maintained by the continued presentation of viral sequences as MHC–peptide complexes.

Pathology of arenavirus infections: general features

The mechanisms by which arenaviruses cause disease in man are not fully understood. There is no evidence that either immunopathological or allergenic processes play any part in causing disease; it appears to be more likely that the disease is caused by direct damage of cells by the virus. Post-mortem studies on patients who died from Junín virus infection have shown generalised lymphadenopathy, endothelial swelling in the capillaries and arterioles of almost every organ, accompanied by a depletion of lymphocytes in the spleen. The virus first replicates in lymphoid tissue, from whence it invades the reticuloendothelial system and those cells concerned in the humoral and cellular immune responses; the host's defence mechanisms are thus impaired. Fatal illness is invariably associated with capillary damage leading to capillary fragility, haemorrhages and irreversible shock (Johnson et al., 1973). Disseminated intravascular coagulation is not a typical feature. Although Lassa fever is often regarded as being hepatotropic, the extent of hepatic damage is insufficient to account for the severity of the clinical disease and serum transaminase values often remain within normal limits except in severe cases. Studies of Lassa virus-infected rhesus monkeys have shown that changes in vascular function may play a much greater role in pathogenesis, as a result either of viral replication in the vascular epithelium or secondary effects of virus activity in different organs. Platelet and epithelial cell functions fail immediately before death and are accompanied by a drop in the level of prostacyclin; these functions rapidly return to normal in animals surviving infection (Fisher-Hoch et al., 1987). Impairment of the functions of vascular epithelium in the absence of histological changes appears to be a common feature of the final stages of viral haemorrhagic diseases in general and suggests that hypovolaemic shock may be amenable to treatment with prostacyclin.

The pathogenesis of Argentine haemorrhagic fever has been studied in guinea pigs infected with Junín virus, this being a suitable model of human disease. There is a pronounced thrombocytopenia and leucopenia characteristic of human infections, and animals die of severe haemorrhagic lesions. Bone marrow cells are destroyed with the release of proteases and acid and alkaline phosphatases into the blood; this leads to consumption of the C4 complement component. These effects may lead in turn to progressive alterations in vascular permeability and platelet function (Rimoldi and de Bracco, 1980). The most extensive histopathological studies have been made on tissues from patients with Lassa fever (Walker and Murphy, 1987). However, there are many similarities in the pathological lesions found in man following Junín and Machupo virus infections. Focal non-zonal necrosis in the liver has been described in all three conditions with hyperplasia of Kupffer cells, erythrophagocytosis and acidophilic necrosis of hepatocytes. Councilman-like bodies can be observed together with cytoplasmic vacuolations and nuclear pyknosis or lysis. As with other organs, there is little evidence of cellular inflammation. Lesions in other organs have been described, including interstitial pneumonitis, tubular necrosis in kidney, lymphocytic infiltration of spleen and minimal inflammation of central nervous system and myocardium (Walker and Murphy, 1987). The hepatic changes may range from mild, focal necrosis to extensive zonal necrosis involving up to 50% of hepatocytes. These changes are consistent with a direct cytolytic action of the virus; nevertheless, the simultaneous presence of Lassa virus and specific antibodies during the later stages of the acute disease suggests that antibody-dependent cellular immune reactions may also occur. Microscopic changes in the kidneys are minimal, although it is not clear whether the functional impairment is due to the deposition of antigen–antibody complexes.

Lymphocytic choriomeningitis

Clinical and pathological features

Infection is often inapparent but may present as an influenza-like febrile illness, as aseptic meningitis or, rarely, as severe meningoencephalomyelitis. The great majority of LCM virus infections are, however, benign. The incubation period is 6–13 days. In the influenza-like illness there is fever, malaise, muscular pains and bronchitis. An early leucopenia followed by lymphocytosis is a constant finding. Generally, the mean value of mononuclear cells is approximately 600 cells/mm^3, although counts of up to 3000 mm^{-3} have been recorded. A coryza together with retro-orbital pain, anorexia and nausea are common. During the acute phase a large number of mononuclear cells are present in the cerebrospinal fluid (CSF) as part of a pleocytosis, although the absolute number varies with time after onset.

As with all central nervous system diseases, the CSF is at increased pressure, with a slight rise in protein concentration, normal or slightly reduced sugar concentration, and a moderate number of cells, mainly lymphocytes ($150-400$ mm^{-3}). It has been noted that the majority of such patients have a history of influenza-like illness immediately prior to the onset of meningitis. The meningeal form is more common; the same symptoms may remain mild and be of short duration and patients recover within a few days, but there can be a more pronounced illness with severe prostration lasting 2 weeks or more. Chronic sequelae have been reported on occasion, including parotitis and orchitis. Other symptoms include continuing headache, paralysis and personality changes. The few deaths reported have followed severe meningoencephalomyelitis. In this most severe form, patients may rapidly develop a bilateral papilloedema, confusion and paralysis of the extremities over a 1-week period. An erythematous rash followed by haemorrhage and death has also been reported. Virus can be isolated from blood, CSF and, in fatal cases, from brain tissue. However, the preferred method of diagnosis is antibody detection by immunofluorescence, although the test is not readily available in most clinical virology laboratories. Because of the possible diagnosis of related, more hazardous arenaviruses, it cannot be stressed too often that samples should be referred to an internationally recognised reference laboratory.

Epidemiology

Man is usually infected through contact with rodents. In the past, these infections have been most often acquired in laboratories, where LCM may be a contaminant in laboratory colonies of mice and hamsters. In particular, virus is shed from the urine of persistently infected animals, resulting in contamination of skin and working surfaces. Hamsters kept as pet animals have also played a role in human infection. The mechanism of transmission of the virus to man is not fully understood but is likely to involve dust contaminated by urine, the contamination of food and drink, or via skin abrasions.

A number of studies have shown evidence of LCM virus infection in human populations, both urban and rural. Seroprevalence rates in the range of $2-5\%$ have been reported from regions as far apart as Nova Scotia in Canada (Marrie and Saron, 1998) and in Santa Fe province, Argentina (Ambrosio et al., 1994). A more recent study by Lledo and colleagues (2003) centred on Madrid showed a significantly higher rate in females, a feature also of the Nova Scotian study. The reasons for this are obscure, although if confirmed could be of importance in recognising LCM virus infections among pregnant women, especially given the potential teratogenic capacity of this virus. Not surprisingly, LCM virus infection occurs with high frequency among feral *Mus musculus* rodents: these frequencies have been reported as high as 9% in urban areas (Childs et al., 1991). Collectively, these findings argue for an increasing awareness for LCM virus among patients presenting with asceptic meningitis or encephalitis.

A variant of LCM virus has been isolated from captive New World primates. The histopathology in infected marmosets and tamarins is remarkably similar to that seen in Lassa virus infection in humans. It is suspected that these animals acquired the virus from infected *M. musculus* rodents (Stephensen et al., 1991; Montali et al., 1995).

Lassa fever

History

In 1969, Lassa virus made a dramatic appearance in Nigeria as a lethal, highly transmissible disease. The first victim was an American nurse who was infected in a small mission station in the Lassa township in northeastern Nigeria, whence the virus and the disease derive their names (Fig. 5). The origin of the infection was never determined, although it is thought to have been acquired through direct contact with an infected patient in Lassa. When the nurse's condition steadily deteriorated she was flown to the Evangel Hospital in Jos, where she died the following day. While she was in hospital she was cared for by two other American nurses, one of whom also became infected by direct contact, probably through skin abrasion. This nurse became unwell after an 8-day incubation period and died following an illness lasting 11 days. The head nurse of the hospital, who has assisted at the post-mortem of the first patient, fell ill 7 days after the death of the second patient for whom she had cared, and from whom she

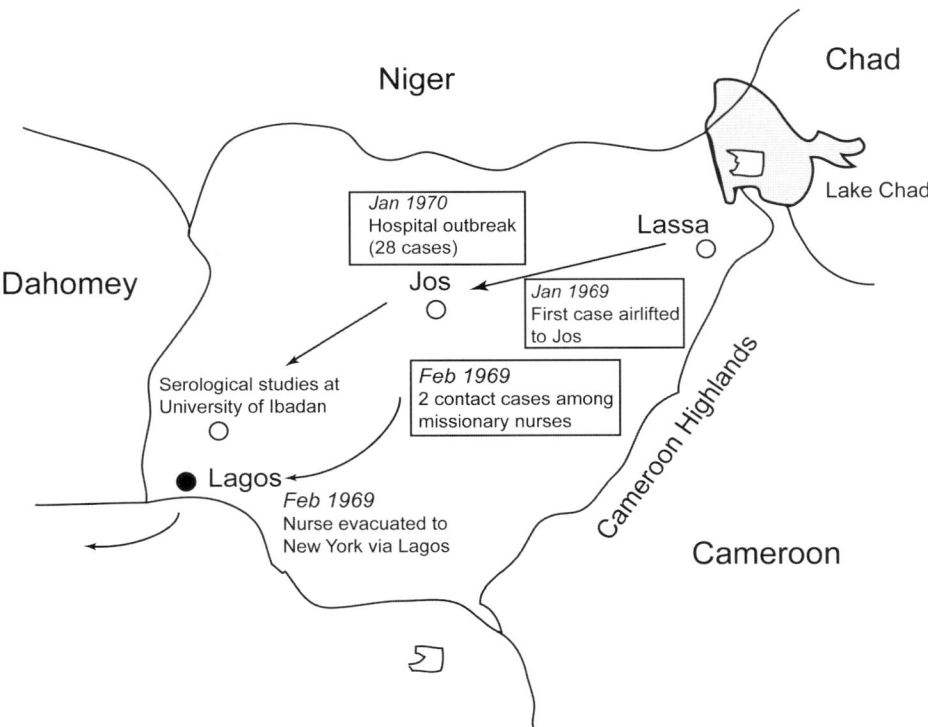

Fig. 5 Map of Nigeria showing the localities of the 1969 and 1970 outbreaks of Lassa fever virus.

probably acquired the infection. This third case was evacuated to the USA by air. After a severe illness under intensive care she slowly recovered. A virus, subsequently named Lassa, was isolated from her blood by workers at the Yale Arbovirus Unit in New Haven, Connecticut. One of these virologists became ill after being exposed to the urine of infected mice. Fortunately his condition improved after a transfusion with immune plasma donated by the third case. Five months after this infection, a laboratory technician in the Yale laboratories, who had not been working with Lassa virus, fell ill and died. The manner in which this infection was acquired has never been determined. This trail of events, not unnaturally, earned for Lassa virus a formidable notoriety, enhanced still further by two more devastating hospital outbreaks—one in Nigeria, the other in Liberia.

A fourth outbreak was seen in Sierra Leone in October 1972. In sharp contrast to the previous outbreaks, this one was not confined to hospitals, although hospital staffs were at considerable risk and several became infected. Most of the patients acquired their illness in the community and there were several intrafamilial transmissions. This led to a revision of the initial view—formed from experience of nosocomial infections—that Lassa fever has a high mortality.

Lassa fever has since continued to occur in West Africa, usually as sporadic cases (Monath, 1987). Between 1969 and 1978 there were 17 reported outbreaks affecting 386 patients, in whom the mortality was 27%. Eleven of the episodes were in hospitals, where the case fatality rate reached 44%; two were laboratory infections, and four acquired in the local community. Eight patients were flown to Europe or North America. One of them was evacuated with full isolation precautions and the remainder, of whom five were infectious, travelled on scheduled commercial flights as fare-paying passengers. Fortunately, no contact cases resulted.

Clinical features

Lassa virus causes a spectrum of disease ranging from the sub-clinical to a fulminating, fatal infection. Studies in Sierra Leone show that most patients present with only a mild form of the disease and this resolves with good primary healthcare. The incubation period ranges from 3 to 16 days and the illness usually begins insidiously. The disease is difficult to distinguish in the early stages from other systematic febrile illnesses, most notably malaria, septicaemia and yellow fever. The most reliable clinical signs on presentation are a sore throat, myalgia, abdominal and lower back pains, accompanied by vomiting. Occasionally a faint maculopapular rash may be seen during the second week of illness on the face, neck, trunk and arms. Cough is a common symptom, and light-headedness, vertigo and tinnitus appear in a few patients. The fever generally lasts 7–17 days and is variable. Convalescence begins in the second to fourth weeks, when the temperature returns to normal and the symptoms improve. Most patients complain of extreme fatigue for several weeks. Loss of hair is common and deafness afflicts one in four patients, and there may be brief bouts of fever.

In a significant number of cases the symptoms suddenly worsen after the first week, with continuing high fever, severe prostration, chest and abdominal pains, conjunctival injection, diarrhoea, dysphagia and vomiting. One important physical finding is a distinct pharyngitis; yellow-white exudative spots may be seen on the tonsillar pillars together with small vesicles and ulcers. The patient appears toxic, lethargic and dehydrated; the blood pressure is low and there is sometimes a bradycardia relative to the body temperature. Not uncommonly, patients in whom the disease is eventually fatal have a high-sustained fever. There may be cervical lymphadenopathy, an encephalopathy, and coated tongue, puffiness of the face and neck, and blurred vision. In approximately 25% of cases there is marked involvement of the CNS, manifested by disorientation, ataxia and seizures. Progression to severe haemorrhaging occurs in around a fifth of patients and it is among such patients that mortality exceeds 50%. Death is due to shock, anoxia, respiratory insufficiency and cardiac arrest. Lassa fever is particularly severe in pregnant women. A study of 75 women in Sierra Leone showed that 11 of 14 deaths were the result of infection during the third trimester; a further 23 patients suffered abortion in the first and second trimesters.

Epidemiology

Lassa virus is endemic in Nigeria and the West Africa states of Guinea, Sierra Leone and Liberia. Outbreaks occur regularly, for example in the 12 years between 1996 and 1997 over 1000 cases were recorded in Sierra Leone with 148 deaths. The situation in the intervening sub-Saharan region is unclear, more likely due to the lack of extensive surveys rather than an absence of infection. Occasional cases have been reported in travellers: a fatal case occurred in a student returning to Germany after having visited Côte d'Ivoire and Ghana before falling ill on his return to Europe (Gunther et al., 2000).

Interestingly Lassa virus appears to be absent from Central Africa. Gonzalez and associates (1989) have suggested that the ecological niche occupied by arenaviruses non-pathogenic for humans is absent, the Cameroon Highlands providing a natural barrier from West Africa where endemic Lassa virus occurs from Nigeria westwards to Sierra Leone.

Nigerian isolates show considerable phylogentic diversity, suggesting Lassa virus has been endemic in the *Mastomys* population of this area for some considerable time. Isolates from Sierra Leone and Liberia form a distinct but closely related lineage, indicating that Lassa virus spread to this region relatively recently, either by migration of persistently infected rodents or by some form of transport. Bowen et al. (2000) have conducted a comparative analysis of 54 West African isolates, both from human cases and from rodents. This study showed a direct linkage between viruses circulating in *Mastomys* and human cases. As with the study of Junín virus isolates from Argentina from cases spanning several decades, there was no evidence of a molecular clock operating (Garcia et al., 2000). This strongly favours the view that arenavirus variation is a function of geography rather than time.

Valuable longitudinal studies have been conducted in Sierra Leone. These revealed that as many as 13% of *all* admissions to two study hospitals were attributable to Lassa virus infections. The highest numbers presented during the dry months from February to May, possibly when rodent numbers are greatest.

Lassa virus has been repeatedly isolated from the multimammate rat *M. natalensis* in Sierra Leone and Nigeria. This rodent is a common domestic and peridomestic species, and large populations are widely distributed in Africa, south of the Sahara. During the rainy season it may desert the open fields and seek shelter indoors. Some genetic variation has been shown in *Mastomys* populations inhabiting different ecological niches; however, there appears to be no difference in the prevalence of antibody and virus in at least two of the karyotypes found in West Africa.

Rodents are infected *in utero* and remain persistently infected for life, secreting about $3-4 \log_{10}$ of virus per ml of urine (McCormick et al., 1987c). Those houses sheltering greater numbers of rodents show a correlation with the seroprevalence of Lassa antibodies among the occupants of such dwellings. Although the average number of infected rodents per household is in single figures, this level of virus excretion presents ample opportunity for human infection as a result of repeated close contact with contaminated surfaces, utensils and foodstuffs. In many areas, the trapping and cooking of rodents is common practice, further escalating the risk of infection. Although virus may be carried on dust, there is little evidence of infection resulting from inhalation of dust particles (Salvato et al., 1992)

Studies of the ratio of clinical illness to infections have confirmed that Lassa fever is endemic in several regions of West Africa. It has been estimated that only 1–2% of infections are fatal–substantially less than the figures of 30–50% originally associated with the early nosocomial outbreaks. However, there may still be up to 300,000 infections per year with as many as 5000 deaths (McCormick et al., 1986b). The seroconversion rates among villagers in Sierra Leone vary from 4–22 per 100 susceptible individuals per year; up to 14% of febrile illness in such population groups is due to Lassa virus infection. There is a marked variation as to the severity of the disease according to different geographical regions. This may in part be due to genotypic variation of Lassa virus, or dose and route of infection, or a combination of these factors (Fisher-Hoch 1993). There is a relatively high rate of asymptomatic and mild infections in endemic areas. One reason for this may be the frequency of re-infections; although about 6% of the population lose antibody annually, rises in antibody titre are also often observed. It is not clear if re-infection results in clinical disease. A finding of incomplete immunity after infection to any significant degree would have profound implications for the use of a vaccine.

There may be secondary spread from person to person in conditions of overcrowded housing and among patients in rural hospitals. There is a particularly high risk to staffs and patients on maternity wards as Lassa fever is a major cause of spontaneous abortion. Medical attendants or relatives who provide direct personal care are most likely to contract the infection; as noted above, accidental inoculation with a sharp instrument and contact with blood have caused infection in a few cases. Airborne spread may take place, as well as mechanical transmission. Although in Sierra Leone there has been no evidence of airborne spread in hospital outbreaks, one of the 1970 outbreaks in Nigeria is believed to have been caused by airborne transmission from a woman with severe pulmonary infection.

Lassa fever is a major cause of spontaneous abortion in West Africa. The virus is readily recovered from the blood and placenta of aborted foetuses. Women generally recover quickly after such abortions, showing a dramatic decline in viraemia, partially due to massive bleeding at the time of abortion (A. Demby, personal communication). Paediatric Lassa fever is known to occur more commonly in male children for unknown reasons. Presenting as an acute febrile illness, the case fatality rate may approach 30% in children with widespread oedema, abdominal distension and bleeding.

Diagnosis

It is important to note that serodiagnosis and virus isolation should be attempted only in laboratories equipped to provide maximum containment to protect the investigator (Biosafety level P4). Suspected cases should be reported immediately to local and national public health authorities prior to any attempt to handle specimens.

The diagnosis of Lassa fever is confirmed by isolation of the virus or demonstration of a specific serological response. Infection in the early stages can be confused clinically with a number of other infectious diseases, particularly malignant malaria (Table 3) (Woodruff, 1975). The two most reliable prognostic markers of fatal infections are the titres of circulating virus and of aspartate aminotransferase (AST). Patients in whom the titre of virus exceeds 10^4 $TCID_{50}$/ml accompanied by AST levels above 150 IU have a poor prognosis, and fatality rates approach 80%. In contrast, patients with virus and enzyme levels below these values have a greater than 85% chance of survival (Johnson et al., 1987). This demonstration of an association between the degree of viraemia and mortality is unique for virus infections and contrasts with the difficulty in predicting the outcome in patients with Argentine and Bolivian haemorrhagic fevers. Although Lassa

Table 3

Differential diagnosis of arenavirus haemorrhagic fevers

Viral disease
Yellow fever
Dengue haemorrhagic fever
Hantavirus

Bacterial disease
Bacterial septicaemia with disseminated intravascular coagulation
Enteric fevers (typhoid, paratyphoid)
Streptococcal pharyngitis
Typhus

Parasitic disease
Trypanosomiasis
Malaria
Leptospirosis

fever can be diagnosed accurately from the presence of IgM antibodies on admission, there is no correlation between the time of appearance, the titre of specific antibodies and clinical outcome.

Lassa virus grows readily in Vero cell culture and virus can usually be isolated within 4 days. Virus can be cultured from serum, throat washings, pleural fluid and urine; it is excreted from the pharynx for up to 14 days after the onset of illness and in urine for up to 67 days after onset. Lassa infection can be diagnosed early by detection of virus-specific antigens in conjunctival cells using indirect immunofluorescence. The use of RT-PCR method is possible, although these techniques are of limited practical use in endemic areas.

The most sensitive serological test for the detection of Lassa antibodies is indirect immunofluorescence; antibodies can be detected by this method in the second week of illness. Complement-fixing antibodies develop more slowly and are rarely detectable before the third week after onset. On occasions, complement-fixing antibodies failed to develop in patients from whom Lassa virus has been isolated. Neutralising antibodies are difficult to measure *in vitro*, in sharp contrast to infections by the South American arenaviruses, for reasons that are unclear.

Therapy

Although the passive administration of Lassa immune plasma may suppress viraemia and favourably alter the clinical outcome, it does not always do so, particularly if the patient has a high virus burden (McCormick et al., 1986c). Failure may be due to the difficulty in assessing accurately the titre of viral neutralising antibodies in the plasma, the late and non-uniform nature of this response in convalescence, and antigenic variation. The widespread occurrence of human immunodeficiency virus (HIV) infections in West Africa precludes at present the use of immune plasma from convalescent individuals in this region. This is in marked contrast to the benefit of immune plasma in the treatment of Junín infections. This may be due either to the high titre of neutralising antibodies that develops soon after the acute phase or to the lesser importance of antibody in the resolution of Lassa virus.

Greater success has been achieved with antivirals. In one study of patients with a poor prognosis, treatment for 10 days with intravenous ribavirin (60–70 mg/kg per day) within 6 days after the onset of fever showed a case fatality rate reduced to 5% (McCormick et al., 1986a). In contrast, patients treated 7 or more days after the onset of fever had a case fatality rate of 26%. In the Sierra Leone study, viraemia of greater than $10^{3.6}$ TCID$_{50}$/ml on admission was associated with a case fatality rate of 76%. Patients with this risk factor who were treated with intravenous ribavirin within 6 days of the onset of fever had a case fatality rate of 9% compared with 47% among those treated 7 days or more after the onset of illness. Oral ribavirin is less effective. A difficulty with its use, however, is that ribavirin can induce haemolytic anaemia in over 40% of patients.

The introduction of vaccines against Junín virus has stimulated the expectation that a vaccine could also be developed for the prevention of Lassa virus infections. Certainly the disease burden in West Africa plus the risk to travellers would warrant the availability of a vaccine but this is unlikely to come from the private sector. Attempts to produce a vaccine against Lassa fever have not as yet progressed beyond experimental challenge studies in guinea pigs and non-human primates. Both the nucleoprotein N and the envelope glycoproteins expressed by vaccinia constructs protect guinea pigs against challenge with Lassa virus, but these encouraging results did not translate into successful protection of primates, with only the glycoprotein construct conferring protection (Morrison et al., 1989). However, there did not appear to be any correlation between antibody titre and resistance to live virus challenge. Taken together with the finding that inactivated Lassa virus also failed to protect primates despite high levels of anti-Lassa antibodies, it appears a significant class I MHC-restricted cytotoxic T cell response is necessary in order to limit virus replication. There is circumstantial evidence from human studies also suggesting antibodies are often present at the time of presentation, but the presence of antibodies does not correlate with disease severity or outcome. Bausch et al. (2000) have gone as far as suggesting that the presence of anti-N antibodies may actually be a poor predictor of outcome. All this contrasts markedly with the outstanding success of Argentine clinicians in treating cases of Junín infection with immune plasma, and the encouraging results that have been obtained with the "Candidate 1" Junín virus vaccine.

A rigorous study in rhesus monkeys sheds light on the difficulties in producing a Lassa virus vaccine (Fisher-Hoch et al., 2000). Immunisation of primates with vaccinia virus expressing all of the S RNA gene products survived challenge with $10^3 - 10^4$ pfu of virus. Animals receiving one or other of the glycoproteins GP1 and GP2 died but those that received both GP1 and GP2 delivered at separate sites survived, despite the fact that anti-GP1/GP2 antibodies could not be detected prior to live virus challenge. Anti-nucleocapsid (N) antibodies, in contrast, had no protective effect. Although these data are encouraging, it needs to be remembered that none of these immunogens actually prevented replication of the challenge virus, an observation that could well restrain any attempts at performing clinical trials in humans. The work of Yang et al. clearly shows that antibody can play an important role in protection, although a substantial CTL response is most likely necessary for control of virus replication (Table 4).

Control

Containment of Lassa fever virus depends upon the strict isolation of cases, rigorous disinfection, rodent control and effective surveillance. Nosocomial transmission presents a considerable risk and patient isolation—in isolators when available—is an absolute must. Strict procedures for dealing with body fluids and excreta need to be enforced. Disinfection with 0.5% sodium hyperchlorite or 0.5% phenol in detergent is recommended for instruments and surfaces. Given the higher virus burden in cases of Lassa fever compared to patients with Junín or Machupo virus infections, surveillance of those having been in contact with Lassa fever patients is also a high public health priority. WHO recommends that those who have been in non-casual contact with cases should be observed for 3 months after their last contact with the patient. This follow up should consist of taking body temperature measurements twice daily. Infection should be

Table 4

Immunisation of non-human primates with recombinant vaccinia constructs expressing Lassa virus proteins (from Yang et al., 2000)

Group	Viral protein(s)	n	Survivors	Protection (%)	Median day of death	Mean viraemia ($\log_{10}$)
Controls	Vaccinia	3	0	0	15	5.7
	None	7	0	0	12	
Single glycoprotein	G1	2	0	0	15	6.8
	G2	2	0	0	12.5	
Nucleoprotein	N	11	3	27	11.5	6.7
Full glycoprotein	G	7	6	86	21	2.5
	G1 + G2	2	2	100		
Full S segment	Mopeia virus	2	2	100		
	G + N	6	5	83	11	7.0
	N	2	2	100		
Total		44	20	90		

suspected if the body temperature exceeds 38.3°C (101°F) and the contact hospitalised immediately.

Rodent control is frequently difficult, although much can be done to minimise contact by isolating foodstuffs, preventing rodent entry into dwellings, and reducing the chance of inhabitants coming into contact with rodent excreta.

The South American haemorrhagic fevers

Diagnosis of Bolivian and Argentine haemorrhagic fevers

Although the clinical features of Bolivian and Argentine haemorrhagic fevers are similar, the laboratory diagnosis of these diseases is approached in a somewhat different manner. In the case of Junín, virus can be recovered consistently from the blood from the 3rd to the 8th day of illness; in contrast, direct recovery of Machupo virus from acutely ill patients is much more difficult, only being recovered from 20% at best from acute phase sera, and even less successfully from urine and throat swabs. Virus cannot be recovered from the CSF of patients with CNS involvement. In both instances, serological methods are more useful.

Complement-fixing antibodies may be detected sufficiently early in both the cases, provided suitable paired sera are available. Although this technique has now largely been superseded by the use of more sensitive immunofluorescence methods and ELISA, the appearance of complement-fixing antibodies has been promoted in the past as providing useful information to the course of the infection and signals the onset of convalescence. Early use of immunofluorescence techniques for the diagnosis of Argentine haemorrhagic fever showed that specific antibodies could be detected by the indirect method approximately 30 days after onset of symptoms. Specific staining is generally seen as a bright, granular fluorescence evenly distributed over the cytoplasm of the fixed infected cell substrate. The titre of immunofluorescent antibodies increases from the 12th to the 20th day of illness with a mixture of IgG and IgM antibodies.

Neutralising antibodies to both Machupo and Junín viruses persist for many years at high titre, appearing simultaneously with complement-fixing antibodies. The sensitivity and specificity of neutralisation tests for detecting immunity to Junín virus has proven to be of value retrospectively in the detection of individuals with sub-clinical infections. The test may be carried out in Vero cell monolayers by varying virus dilution in the presence of a fixed concentration of serum. Antibody titres are then expressed as an index calculated by subtracting the logarithmic differences between the virus titre in the control and experimental reactions. Inapparent infections have been shown in approximately 20% of laboratory workers handling known or presumptively positive specimens by this method.

Argentine haemorrhagic fever (Junín virus)

Epidemiology

Argentine haemorrhagic fever has been known since 1943 and Junín virus, the causative agent, was first isolated in 1958. From what we now know regarding the phylogenetic relationships between arenaviruses, it is clear from anecdotal accounts that arenaviruses have existed for many years in zoonotic foci. Marr and Kiracofe (2000) have suggested that arenaviruses may have even contributed to the downfall of the indigenous Mexican population in the 16th century. Records tell of a "great pestilence" afflicting Spaniards, African and the local population alike. Argentine haemorrhagic fever has a marked seasonal incidence over an area approximately 150,000 km^2, coinciding with the maize harvest between April and July, when rodent populations reach their peak (Fig. 6). The incidence tends to be greatest in newly affected areas, followed by a decline in attack rates in the years that follow. Increasing herd immunity, fluctuations in rodent number, and changing agricultural practice may individually, or in combination, account for swings in the incidence of infection from year to year. Person-to-person transmission has not been observed, probably due to the relatively low titre of circulating virus. The endemic zone has expanded progressively northwards and eastwards from the Pampas region of Argentina to the extent that now some 5 million people are at risk, approximately 1 in 5 of the total Argentine population (Maiztegui et al., 1986).

Agricultural workers, particularly those harvesting maize, are, not surprisingly, the most commonly affected. The main reservoir hosts of Junín virus are *Calomys* field voles that live and breed in burrows under the maize fields and in the surrounding grass banks (Fig. 7). Other rodent species may also be infected. *Calomys* spp. have a persistent viraemia and viruria, and the virus is also present in considerable quantities in the saliva. The mode of transmission of Junín virus to man has not been conclusively established. The virus may be carried in the air or dust contaminated by rodent excreta or may enter by

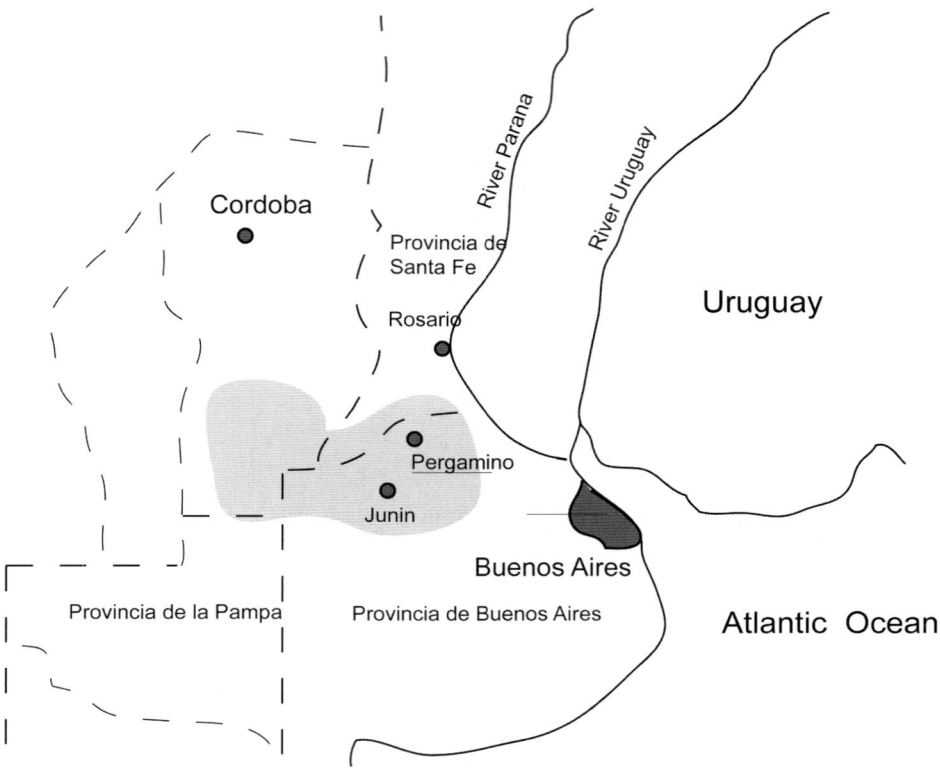

Fig. 6 Approximate endemic zone of Argentine haemorrhagic fever.

ingestion of contaminated foodstuffs. Recent phylogenetic analyses have separated isolates into three distinct clades that equate with a strong geographical clustering of cases. This clustering is not related in any obvious way to changes in pathogenicity or virulence, however.

Clinical and pathological features

The virus causes annual outbreaks of severe illness, with between 100 and 800 cases, in an area of intensive agriculture known as the wet pampas in Argentina. The majority of the infections occur in adult male agricultural workers, although cases do occur in all age groups and in both sexes all year round. Operators of agricultural machinery are particularly at risk. Mortality in some outbreaks has ranged from 10 to 20%, although the overall mortality is generally 3–15%. After an incubation period of 7–16 days, the onset

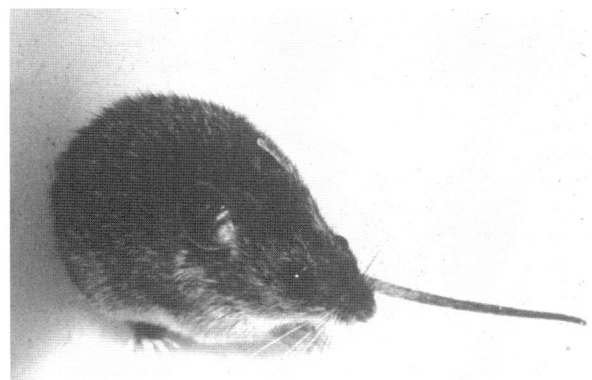

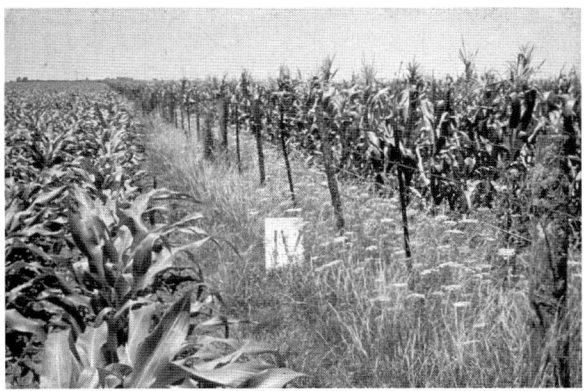

Fig. 7 The habitat for the rodent *Calomys* spp. in the wet pampas of Argentina (from Howard, 1986).

of illness is insidious, with chills, headache, malaise, myalgia, retro-orbital pain and nausea; these symptoms are followed by fever, conjunctival injection and suffusion, a pharyngeal enanthema and erythema and oedema of the face, neck and upper thorax. A few petechiae may be seen, mostly in the axilla. There is hypervascularity and occasional ulceration of the soft palate. Generalised lymphadenopathy is common. Tongue tremor is an early sign, and some patients present with pneumonitis. Sub-clinical infections do occur. In the more severe cases the patient's condition becomes appreciably worse after a few days, with the development of hypotension, oliguria, haemorrhages from the nose and gums (Fig. 8), haematemesis, haemtauria and melaena. Oliguria may progress to anuria and pronounced neurological manifestations may develop. Laboratory findings have included leucopenia WBC count (<2500 mm^{-3}) with a decrease in the number of CD4 positive cells, thromobocytopenia ($<100,000$ mm^{-3}) and urinary casts containing viral antigen. Patients recover when the fever falls, followed by diuresis and rapid improvement. Death may result from hypovolaemic shock.

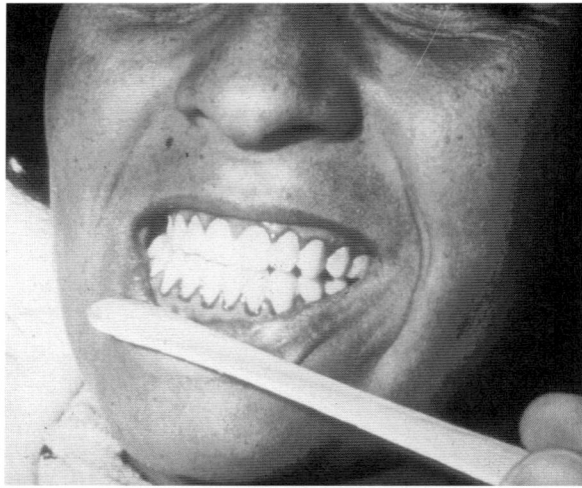

Fig. 8 Bleeding from the gum margin in a case of Argentine haemorrhagic fever (from Howard, 1986).

Therapy

In contrast to Lassa fever, antibodies play a major role in recovery from Junín infection. Controlled trials of immune plasma collected from patients at least 6 months into convalescence have shown a dramatic reduction in mortality if plasma is given within the first 8 days of illness (Maiztegui et al., 1979). The efficacy of this therapy is directly related to the titre of neutralising antibody in the plasma; as a result a dose of no less than 3000 "therapeutic units"/kg body weight has been recommended (Enria et al., 1984). The late development of a neurological syndrome is seen in up to 10% of patients treated with immune plasma; it is often benign and self-limiting but points to the possible persistence of viral antigens on cells of the central nervous system well into convalescence. Treatment with immune plasma also restores the response of peripheral blood lymphocytes to antigenic stimuli, suggesting that administration of plasma also results in the modulation of cellular immunity.

A small trial of ribavirin involving 18 patients has been reported by Huggins et al. (1989). The mortality was 12.5% in those receiving interferon compared with 40% among the controls. However, a more thorough study using larger patient numbers has not been conducted.

Prophylaxis

There have been several attempts to produce a vaccine against Argentine haemorrhagic fever. The XJC1$_3$ strain of virus grown in the brains of suckling mice is relatively non-pathogenic and was administered to 636 volunteers between 1968 and 1970. Over a period of 3 years, 70 cases of Junín virus infection occurred among the population but there were no cases amongst those immunised. However, the vaccine often induced a mild febrile reaction or a subclinical infection, and its use was discontinued despite the fact that over 90% of vaccinees maintained neutralising antibody for up to 9 years. There have been renewed attempts during recent years to develop a new vaccine strain sufficiently attenuated for human use and meeting modern day requirements as to derivation, manufacture and potency. Several clones have been prepared in foetal rhesus lung cells from the original XJ isolate, one of which exhibits less neurovirulence than the XJCl₃ strain and yet protected rhesus monkeys against challenge with wild type Junín virus (McKee et al., 1993). This "Candidate 1" vaccine has been tested in a double-blind study in volunteers (Maiztegui et al., 1998). A total of 6500 male agricultural workers were recruited to the randomised, double-blind controlled study over a 2-year period. A total of 23 males developed Argentine haemorrhagic fever, all but one having received the vaccine. A further three mild cases were seen in both the vaccinated and unvaccinated cohorts, giving a vaccine efficacy of 95% for preventing clinical illness and 84% efficacy against infection. Unconfirmed reports suggest that immunity lasts at least 3 years.

Bolivian haemorrhagic fever (Machupo virus)

Clinical features

Bolivian haemorrhagic fever was first recognised in 1959 in the Beni region in north-eastern Bolivia with 470 reported cases in the years up to 1962. The disease continued in that region more or less annually for a number of years in the form of sharply localised epidemics, most commonly between April and July coinciding—as with Argentine haemorrhagic fever—with the annual harvest. Its incidence has decreased considerably since the late 1960s and human infections are now rarely reported. It is worth noting that the discovery of a common morphology and serological cross-reaction between Machupo and LCM virus led to the concept of the arenavirus family. The mortality in individual outbreaks varied from 5 to 30%. From 1962 to 1964 there was a further series of outbreaks involving upwards of 1000 patients with 180 deaths. The most notable outbreak affected 700 people in the San Joaquin township between late 1962 and the middle of 1964. The mortality was 18%. After a break of some 20 years, fresh outbreak occurred in 1994 in north-eastern Bolivia involving 19 cases, with at least seven deaths, six in a single family in the town of Magdelana, the latter cluster almost certainly the result of secondary spread from an index case of naturally acquired infection. These were the first recorded since 1971; for reasons that are obscure, this outbreak did not appear linked to any major changes in rodent numbers or behaviour. A further eight cases were reported in 1999 and 18 in 2000, suggesting that Machupo virus infection may be increasing in activity once more.

The clinical disease is similar to Argentine haemorrhagic fever. The incubation period ranges from 7 to 14 days and the onset is insidious, beginning with an influenza-like illness accompanied by malaise and fatigue. This is followed by abdominal pain, anorexia, tremors, prostration and severe limb pain. About one-third of patients show a tendency to bleed, with petechiae on the trunk and palate, and bleeding from the gastrointestinal tract, nose, gums and uterus. Almost half the patients develop a fine tremor of the tongue and hands, and some may have more pronounced neurological symptoms. The acute disease may last 2–3 weeks and convalescence may be protracted, generalised weakness being the most common complaint. Clinically inapparent infections are rare. Machupo virus, the responsible agent, is readily isolated from both lymph nodes and spleen taken at autopsy. Isolation of the virus from acutely ill patients has proved difficult, however, the best results being obtained from specimens taken 7–12 days after the onset of illness.

Epidemiology

The rodent reservoir of Machupo virus is the field vole *Calomys callosus* that can frequent dwellings and outhouses; over 60% of animals caught during the San Joaquin epidemic were found to be infected. Virus is shed in the saliva, urine and faeces of infected animals. The distribution of cases in San Joachin was associated with certain houses and *C. callosus* was trapped in all households where cases occurred. Transmission to man is probably by contamination of food and water or by infection through skin abrasions. Transmission from man to man is unusual but a small episode took place in 1971, well outside the endemic zone. The index case, infected in Beni, carried the infection to Cochabamba and, by direct transmission, caused five secondary cases, of which four were fatal.

Abnormally low rainfall, combined with an increase in the use of insecticide, led to a rapid decline in the numbers of cats, with the result that the population of Machupo-infected rodents increased dramatically, thus increasing the opportunity for human contact with contaminated soil and foodstuffs. This balance has since been restored, consistent with the decline in the number of reported cases over the past two decades.

Treatment

As with AHF, treatment is largely supportive. Although attempts have been made to use convalescent immune plasma from survivors of Machupo infection, a combination of a lack of facilities in Bolivia suited to the treating of collected plasma and the absence of a controlled trial as to the efficacy of its use means that the treatment of patients with immunoglobulin remains speculative. Intravenous ribavirin was administered to two patients during the 1994 outbreak (Kilgore et al., 1997): both the patients recovered but in the absence of carefully controlled clinical trials there is no certain indication that ribavirin is effective against Machupo infection.

Brazilian haemorrhagic fever (Sabiá virus)

This arenavirus was isolated in 1990 from human cases at autopsy (Lisieux et al., 1994). The source of this infection was uncertain but is likely to have been acquired by exposure to infected rodents in an agricultural setting in an area immediately outside São Paulo. As a continuing reminder of the potential severity of these infections, a laboratory worker became critically ill after having been accidentally exposed to an aerosol containing Sabiá virus. The virus was first isolated from a fatal case of haemorrhagic fever. A laboratory-acquired infection was characterised by a febrile illness accompanied by leucopaenia and thrombocytopenia. There is little information regarding the epidemiology of this virus, although the extensive liver necrosis seen in the first case is a warning that this and other haemophagic fevers may on first examination be mistaken for yellow fever.

Venezuela haemorrhagic fever (Guanarito virus)

Between May 1990 and March 1991 an outbreak occurred among residents of Guanarito municipality on the central plains of Venezuela. Originally mistaken for dengue fever, a total of 104 cases were recorded with a mortality rate of around 25%. The Guanarito virus was subsequently isolated from the spleens of such cases at autopsy. The disease has appeared in subsequent years between November and January, occurring predominantly among male agricultural workers (de Manzione et al., 1998). A further outbreak occurred in 2002 involving more than 20 cases. The principal rodent hosts of this virus have been identified (Table 1) (Tesh et al., 1994). The outbreaks appear to have been the consequence of forest clearance to make way for agricultural land, this providing ample breeding grounds for the carrier, the cane mouse *Zygodontomys brevicauda*.

The disease has a clinical profile similar to that of Argentine haemorrhagic fever, with patients manifesting thrombocytopenia, haemorrhaging and neurological signs. There are distinct differences, however, compared to the haemorrhagic diseases caused by other South American arenaviruses. Diarrhoea and pharyngitis are more common and deafness reported in convalescent patients. Although initial reports suggest a high mortality for this infection, antibody prevalence rates of up to 3% have been found among healthy individuals and up to 10% of household contacts have anti-Guanarito virus antibodies.

Emerging arenavirus infections

Oliveros virus

This new agent has been isolated from a small rodent *Bolomys obscurus*, within the endemic region of Argentine haemorrhagic fever (Bowen et al., 1996). With a rodent host distinct from that of Junín virus, approximately 25% of captured *B. obscurus* have been found to contain antibodies to this virus. At present, there are no indications that this virus causes significant numbers of human infections (Mills et al., 1996).

Whitewater Arroyo virus and other isolates from the USA

As a consequence of the 1993 hantavirus outbreak on the Colorado Plateau, there has been intensive study of rodent populations in order to gauge the extent of Sin Nombre Virus distribution and the risk that infected rodents present to rural populations in the USA. During one such study, Kosoy et al. (1996) found an unexpectedly high level of arenavirus antibodies in pack rats (*Neotoma* spp.) caught in the Whitewater Arroyo of New Mexico. Members of the *Neotoma* family are ubiquitous throughout the southwestern part of the USA. Independently Fulhorst and colleagues (1996) described the isolation of a hitherto unknown arenavirus from trapped examples of *N. albigula*. The importance of these findings became evident when in 1999 and 2000 three female patients residing in California presented with symptoms subsequently ascribed to infection with the same arenavirus. One patient had most likely acquired the virus at home when clearing up rodent droppings. Although there was no obvious link between the three cases, each presented with non-specific febrile symptoms and acute respiratory distress. Two developed lymphopenia and thrombocytopenia, and two also showed signs of liver failure and haemorrhage. All three died within 1–8 weeks of onset. Virus was recovered in one and all three gave PCR products that were 87% identical with Whitewater Arroyo Virus.

Yet further new isolations have been made recently. A virus closely related, but distinct from, Whitewater Arroyo Virus has been isolated from the Californian mouse *Peromyscus californicus*. Infectious virus was recovered from 5 of 27 animals caught in the Santa Ana mountains of southern California, close to the Bear Canyon trailhead. It cannot be ruled out that the tentatively dubbed Bear Canyon Virus represents an additional arenavirus that is yet to be associated with human disease.

Table 5

Arenaviruses—key questions

What is the role, if any, of the host cell ribosomes found within virus particles?
What is the function of the Z protein in virus replication?
Do arenaviruses exist among the rodent populations of Asia?
To what extent do the more recently discovered arenaviruses contribute to the burden of disease in the local population?
Why are some arenaviruses (e.g. Junín, Machupo) readily neutralised by antibodies, but others (e.g. Lassa, Pichindé) are not? And what is the implication of this difference for vaccine development?

Summary

The increasing numbers of human infections due to arenaviruses is beginning to require a greater vigilance on the part of public health workers. Arenavirus aetiology for febrile illnesses in individuals residing in endemic areas should be considered, particularly those who are likely to have come into regular contact with rodents by virtue of their lifestyle or occupation.

Although until recently there has been little or no evidence of human arenavirus infection in North America, Europe and Asia, this situation has changed considerably since a greater awareness of the potential for emerging infections has developed among clinicians and microbiologists, particularly in geographical areas where the last decades have seen clearance of woodland, forest and scrub in advance of extensive changes in agricultural practices. This potential has been augmented by changing or abnormal weather patterns, these serving to promote behavioural, if not also numerical, changes in rodent populations. In the Americas, arenavirus investigations have progressively become interleaved with studies on hantavirus distribution, especially in endemic zones where a particular species of rodent may be infected with either a hantavirus or an arenavirus. The only certainty is that the number of arenaviruses identified hitherto will increase as more become known regarding the natural history of these agents.

Bunyaviruses

The Bunyaviridae is a vast family of over 350 RNA viruses grouped into five genera, one of which (the *Tospovirus*) contains viral pathogens of plants and thus will not be considered further. Viruses belonging to the genera *Hantavirus*, *Nairovirus* and *Phlebovirus* all cause severe haemorrhage disease in humans. Given the vast numbers of viruses in this family, those causing viral haemorrhagic fevers represent a mere fraction, although more are probably awaiting discovery as the list of new members continues to grow. Almost all of the bunyaviruses have been encountered as a result of surveillance in wildlife populations and haematophagous insects. Despite the importance of individual members of this family to public and animal health, the vast majority of bunyaviruses are not recognised as being of either medical or veterinary significance.

For a detailed description of the bunyaviruses, see the chapters in Fields Virology by Schmaljohn and Hooper (Schmaljohn, 2001) and Nichol (Nichol, 2001). Additional clinical virology can be found in Swanepoel (2000). There is now an extensive review literature on hantaviruses. Infections in the New World have been reviewed by Peters (1998) and detailed information on European isolates can be had in the review by Vapalahti et al. (2003). These are complemented by a review on phyogenetic relationships by Plyusnin (2002).

General properties of the bunyaviruses

Classification

The family derives its name from bunyamwera virus, discovered when Dr Jordi Casals and his colleagues at the Yale Arbovirus Laboratory begun using serology to group a number of arthropod-isolated agents. Morphological comparisons together with limited biochemical data soon expanded the Bunyamwera supergroup, as it became known, to include significant causes of human disease, particularly the viruses of the California encephalitis group. These viruses are now included in the genus *Bunyavirus*: no members of this genus have been found as causing haemorrhagic disease (but see discussion regarding Garissa virus, page 109).

Additional genera have been created to accommodate viruses with a similar morphology and a broadly similar genetic organisation. Groupings within genera are still heavily reliant upon serological studies, giving rise to a hierarchy of serogroups, antigenic complexes and subtypes. All bunyaviruses possess a segmented, tripartite genome. In common with all studies of virus variation, genome sequencing has played an increasingly important role in bunyavirus classification, particularly in defining the relationships between members of the *Hantavirus* genus.

Viruses in the general *Bunyavirus*, *Nairovirus* and *Phlebovirus* are capable of replication alternatively in arthropods and vertebrates. Although generally cytolytic in mammalian cells, they cause little cytopathogenicity in arthropod vectors. The implication of this property is that viruses within these genera must recognise distinct cellular receptors on vertebrate and invertebrate cells, as well as have the capacity to replicate at near ambient temperature. Some viruses display a very narrow host range for arthropod vectors, although in part this may reflect the dynamics of virus–host interactions that change according to climate and season. Transovarial and venereal transmission have been demonstrated for a number of mosquito-transmitted bunyaviruses, most notably Rift Valley fever virus, a member of the genus *Phlebovirus*.

Hantaviruses appear exceptional in a number of important respects. The most important differences are the absence of arthropod transmission and that hantaviruses frequently cause persistent infections in susceptible mammalian cells. Originally thought to cause haemorrhagic fever with renal syndrome (HFRS) it is now clear that hantaviruses cause a spectrum of severe disease in humans, particularly what is now referred to as hantavirus pulmonary syndrome (HPS).

Structure

Bunyaviruses are spherical or pleomorphic, enveloped viruses with diameters in the range of 80–120 nm. The surface glycoproteins extend up to 10 nm from the lipid bilayer. The latter is derived most frequently from the cytoplasmic membranes that constitute the Golgi apparatus of the infected cell. The fine structure of bunyavirus particles differs between members of the different genera, particularly in the manner by which the major glycoproteins cluster to form surface peplomers. The inner structure is less well defined: the helical nucleocapsid structures are 2–2.5 nm in diameter and vary in length from 200 to 3000 nm, depending upon which of the three RNA segments is encapsidated. Each of the three RNA genome segments is encapsidated individually, and are circular as a result of $3'$ and $5'$ base pairing of the RNA segments.

Genetic organisation

The viral genome comprises three unique RNA segments, designated L (large), M (medium) and S (small). The M and S RNA segments are approximately equal in size. In contrast, the L RNA of CCHF virus is almost twice the length of that of Hantaan and Rift Valley fever viruses. Most of this additional genetic information is reflected in a much larger gene product with autocatalytic domains located within the extended amino terminal sequence (see below). The terminal nucleotides of each RNA segment are base paired to form non-covalently closed, circular nucleic acid structures. These sequences are conserved among viruses within each genus but are distinct from those viruses in other genera. Such terminal sequences are important in defining the genera. The coding strategy is either negative or ambisense. Negative polarity genomes require synthesis of a positive strand before protein expression can be initiated. Ambisense genome segments are confined to the bunyaviruses and arenaviruses (see page 109); this means that genes on a RNA segment are either of positive or negative polarity.

For all bunyaviruses, the L, M and S genome segments encode, respectively, for the RNA polymerase (L protein), the envelope glycoproteins G1 and G2, and the nucleocapsid protein (N). All are expressed by the formation of virus-complementary sense mRNA. The coding for non-structural proteins differs among viruses of the five genera. Rift Valley fever virus, a member of the *Phlebovirus* genus, codes for a single non-structural protein (NSs) expressed by the S RNA segment whereas hantaviruses do not code for any. CCHF encodes for at least two non-structural proteins that are precursors to the envelope glycoproteins.

Replication

Bunyaviruses replicate in the cytoplasm of infected cells. Entry is by endocytosis followed by fusion of viral and cellular membranes within endosomes. As is the case with all negative strand viruses, there follows a period of transcription using copies of the virus-associated L protein carried into the cell at fusion. Translation of the mRNAs originating from the transcribed L and S RNA segments takes place on ribosomes free in the cytoplasm, whereas mRNAs from the M segment template encoding for the envelope glycoproteins are translated by membrane-associated ribosomes within the endoplasmic reticulum. This allows for the translation of a precursor molecule from the M ORF to be directly inserted into the membranes of the Golgi apparatus as a prelude to virus assembly and maturation. These events are critical to the formation of nascent virus, with co-translational cleavage being required to yield separate and correctly folded Gn and Gc proteins that can then undergo glycosylation. In some cases, a non-structural protein (NSs) is also released.

Thereafter in the replication cycle there follows a period of synthesis and encapsidation of antigenome RNA to serve as templates for genomic or sub-genomic RNA. The sub-genomic RNA helps amplify gene products and, being of positive polarity, can be used efficiently as mRNA. The transcription and replication scheme for gene segments that are either of negative polarity or ambisense is shown in Fig. 1.

Virus-specific mRNA molecules contain host-derived primer sequences at their $5'$ ends and are truncated at the $3'$ termini relative to the template. The viral mRNAs are not polyadenylated.

In common with many other enveloped viruses, bunyaviruses assemble at internal membranes. Uukiniemi virus, together with Hantaan virus, is among the most intensively studied viruses in terms of understanding how enveloped proteins are inserted into cytoplasmic membranes and thence transported to the cell surface. The signal sequences within the envelope glycoproteins are key in enabling virus particle assembly to take advantage of protein trafficking through the cytoplasmic membrane compartments. The bunyavirus polyprotein expressed from the M RNA segment and containing both the Gn and Gc envelope glycoproteins is processed immediately as the mRNA is translated, a signal peptide in the precursor programming insertion into the lumen of the endoplasmic

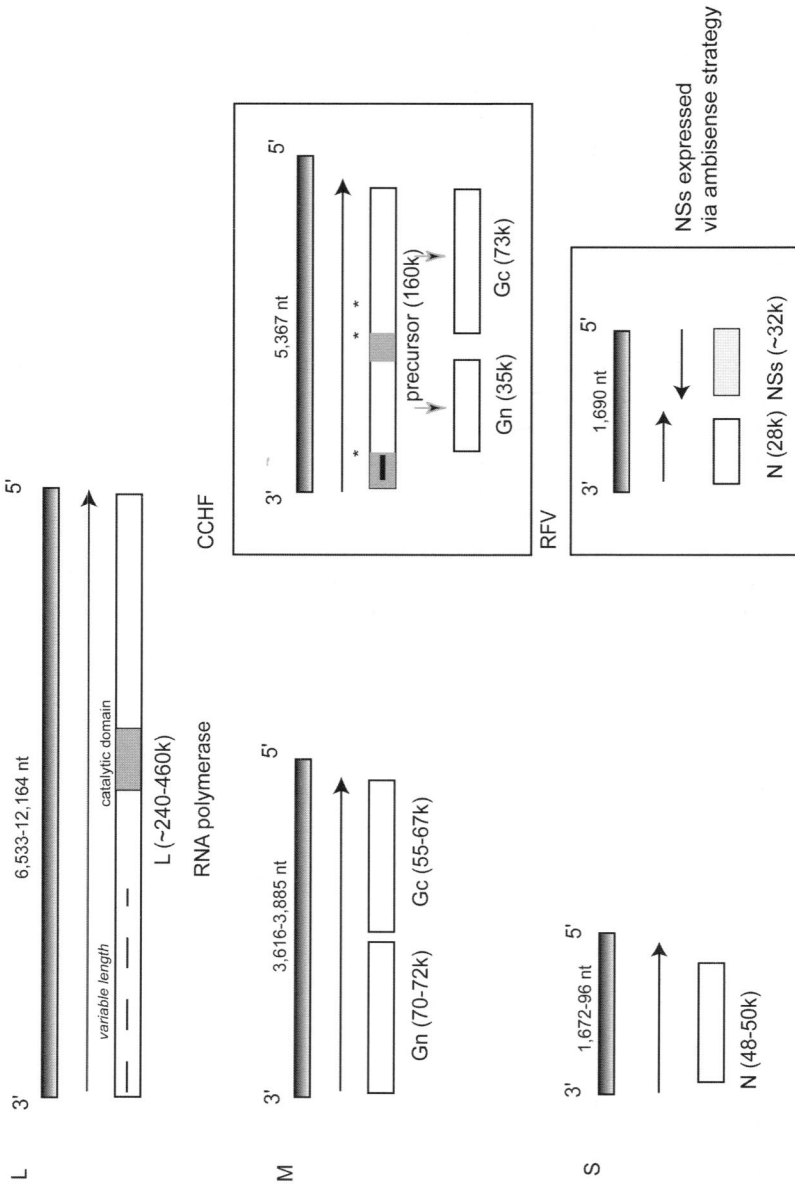

Fig. 1 Genome organisation of the bunyaviruses causing viral haemorrhagic fevers. The L segment codes for the viral RNA polymerase. In the case of CCHF virus, this is almost twice the length, coding for additional sequence at the amino terminus of the L protein which has homology with ovarian tumor (OUT)-like protease and helicase domains. CCHF virus has a unique coding strategy for the M RNA segment; one long precursor molecule with five transmembrane domains is cleaved by host cell proteases (sites marked *) to produce Gn and Gc, respectively. The precursor contains a mucin-like *O*-glycosylated domain at the amino terminus (bar). Rift Valley fever virus produces a shorter N protein from the S RNA segment and an additional, non-structural protein (NSs) via an ambisense coding strategy.

reticulum. A continuing association of Gn and Gc appears necessary for this to happen. Signalling domains in Gn are essential for directing the transport of the maturing surface peplomer and its accumulation in the *cis* or medial compartments.

As with all RNA viruses, the RNA polymerase lacks a proofreading mechanism leading to a high error rate, thus increasing the chance that new antigenic variants will arise. In addition to this process of antigenic drift, the bunyaviruses also have a segmented genome, thus closely related bunyaviruses can exchange segments when dual infection of a single cell occurs. This is more than a theoretical possibility: the newly discovered Garissa virus which has caused cases of haemorrhagic disease in East Africa contains the L and S RNA segments of bunyamwera virus—not a virus normally associated with severe human disease—but a distinct M RNA segment (Bowen et al., 2001).

Crimean-Congo haemorrhagic fever

The virus of Crimean-Congo haemorrhagic fever is a member of the *Nairovirus* genus, named after Nairobi Sheep disease virus. There are seven species with over 30 different strains of variable relationships to each other. These are principally defined by serology owing to a paucity of molecular data, although with the increasing availability of cloned genomes this situation is now changing. Much of the detailed knowledge as to Nairovirus virology comes from the study of Dugbe virus, a Nairovirus that has been isolated many times from ticks across sub-Saharan Africa but appears to have limited capacity for causing human disease. Crimean-Congo haemorrhagic fever is a zoonosis, with human infections the result of either through contact with the blood and carcasses of viraemic animals or by close contact with the ascarid tick vectors responsible for transmission between animals.

Natural history

The virus of Crimean-Congo haemorrhagic fever is widely distributed in Eastern Europe, Africa and Asia, with occasional unconfirmed reports in Western Europe. Crimean-Congo haemorrhagic fever virus has been isolated from over 30 species of hard ticks. In most instances the virus is acquired passively by the imbibing of blood from a viraemic host. The virus appears to replicate only in ixodid ticks, particularly members of the *Hyalomma*, *Dunacentor* and *Rhipicephalus* genera. Species within the *Hyalomma* genus appear particularly important for virus dissemination and there is an overlap between the geographical distributions of *Hyalomma* tick species and the endemic regions of Crimean-Congo haemorrhagic fever.

Hyalomma ticks have a preference for different species of host during their life cycle. Small mammals up to the size of hares are preferred by immature ticks. In contrast, adult ticks associate with larger herbivores: in southern Africa, hosts include wild vertebrates as well as domestic livestock. There have been several reports of transmission from infected to non-infected ticks feeding together on animals that are either not viraemic or immune. This phenomenon of "non-viraemic" transmission between ticks is not unique to Crimean-Congo haemorrhagic fever and has been attributed to factors in tick saliva. Transovarial transmission occurs but at low frequency.

The role of birds in transmission is potentially important, particularly as it has been long recognised that birds migrating between Europe, Asia and Africa can carry transovarially infected immature ticks. Passerine birds and poultry appear not to be susceptible, although ground feeding birds act often as hosts for immature *Hyalomma* ticks.

The greatest risk to humans is exposure to infected blood of sheep, goats and cattle. High prevalence of anti-Crimean-Congo haemorrhagic fever antibodies has been recorded among livestock in areas where *Hyalomma* ticks are common. The virus causes only a mild or inapparent infection in domestic species, but the viraemia is less than the minimum titre needed to infect adult ticks. However, this is almost certainly insufficient to maintain the Crimean-Congo haemorrhagic fever life cycle *per se*, especially as the likelihood of transovarial transmission in ticks is so low. Much more important in maintaining the Crimean-Congo haemorrhagic fever life cycle is infection of immature ticks on small mammals, possibly also on ground feeding birds, such as guinea fowl.

All the evidence suggests that human infections occur through contact of infected blood through skin abrasions and superficial wounds. This agrees with the repeated observation of hospital infections being acquired as a result of accidents with contaminated needles and sharp instruments. The majority of patients tend to be adult males, such as farmers, veterinarians, stockmen and abattoir workers. These predominantly male—and in endemic areas frequently nomadic—individuals thus are exposed whilst carrying out routine husbandry practices such as vaccination, castration and butchering.

Molecular properties

Phylogenetic analyses of the S segment coding for the nucleocapsid (N) protein suggest the existence of at least three genetic subgroups, although there is a proportionally greater sequence diversity in the M RNA segment. It is difficult to correlate such variation with the geographical distribution of the virus, however, due to the random movement of livestock and the international trade in animals that may either harbour infection or be carrying infected ticks (Rodriguez et al., 1997). Different tick hosts may also drive sequence variability, particularly in the envelope glycoproteins. For example, *Hyalomma asiaticum* is the principal host in China as opposed to say, *H. marginatum* in West Africa (Camicas et al., 1994, Yen et al., 1985). Bird migration over long distances may also confound any attempt at locating point source of outbreaks, especially by use of molecular sequencing methods.

A recent study of Chinese isolates collected over a prolonged period from 1966 to 1988 from the Xinjiang Autonomous Region in western China illustrates well these difficulties of interpretation. Sequencing has clearly shown that virus within an epidemic may originate from a variety of sources (Morikawa et al., 2002). This study examined the M RNA segment coding for viral glycoproteins: several isolates were found to cluster with a variant previously isolated in Nigeria. Using highly conserved primers specific for the polymerase gene of the L RNA segment, Honig and associates have reported that the *Nairovirus* genus is highly divergent. Moreover, Honig et al. (2004b) showed a clear phylogenetic lineage for those nairoviruses spread by hard ticks. Thus, Crimean-Congo haemorrhagic fever virus along with other closely related members of the *Nairovirus* genus has evolved closely with their tick hosts.

Examining seven isolates from China, Morikawa et al. (2002) reported that the ORF encoded by the M RNA segment contains a hypervariable region at the N-terminus spanning the first 250 amino acid residues. The location of the N-terminus of Gn within the ORF is still not certain, but Morikawa and colleagues have predicted its location either at residue 1046 or at residue 1054, with some variation between isolates. This locates the cleavage some 50 amino acids downstream of the nearest hydrophobic region towards the end of Gn, similar to that found in the Nairovirus Dugbe. The implication of this is the existence of a common coding strategy for all genes expressed by the M RNA segment, with a non-structural protein located at the N-terminus of the ORF, followed by Gn and Gc, respectively.

A detailed study of the Crimean-Congo haemorrhagic fever virus M RNA products by Sanchez et al. (2002) has extended these findings and more rigorously defined just how Gn and Gc envelope glycoproteins of Crimean-Congo haemorrhagic fever virus are expressed. A cardinal finding by Sanchez and colleagues indicated similarities in glycoprotein processing with viruses of the family Arenaviridae, not just between nairoviruses. Sequencing of the N-termini of Crimean-Congo haemorrhagic fever virus Gn and Gc revealed that the tetrapeptides RRLL and RKPL immediately preceded the Gn and Gc cleavage sites, respectively (Table 1). This same motif has been shown for the Lassa fever virus GPC precursor of the envelope glycoproteins as the recognition site for the cellular protease subtilisin SKI-1/S1P (Lenz et al., 2001). The processing of glycoproteins from a precursor molecule is not found among viruses belonging to other Bunyaviridae genera. A second unexpected finding was that the highly variable N-terminus of the precursor protein possessed features typical of host cell mucins, again a property unique to nairoviruses but found among other viruses causing haemorrhagic disease: for example, the glycoprotein of Ebola virus also possesses a highly variable and richly *O*-glycosylated mucin-like central domain (Sanchez et al., 2002).

The Crimean-Congo haemorrhagic fever L RNA segment codes principally for the viral RNA polymerase. This segment, at 12,164 nucleotides, is almost twice the length of, e.g. that of Rift Valley fever, coding for an L protein of 3944 amino acids as compared to 2149 resides for the L protein of Rift Valley fever virus (Honig et al., 2004a; Kinsella et al., 2004). The increase in size is accounted for by an extension at the N-terminus, this coding for an ovarian tumor (OTU)-like protease. This may have a role in autoproteolysis of this large protein or have a role in its processing through the ubiquination pathway. Other functions are almost certainly represented in this N-terminus sequence, the nature of which is as yet unclear.

Epidemiology

Crimean-Congo haemorrhagic fever virus was first recognised in 1944 among soldiers and agricultural workers in the Crimean Peninsula. Shortly thereafter, filtered

Table 1

The Genus *Hantavirus*: isolates and strains

Virus	Host	Region	Human disease	Comment
Murine associated				
Hantaan	*Apodemus agrarius*	Korea, China, Russia	HFRS/severe	Prototype hantavirus
Dobrava	*Apodemus flavicollis*	Balkans	HFRS/severe	
Saaremaa	*Apodemus agrarius*	Eastern Europe	HFRS/mild	Initially considered a Dobrava variant
Seoul	*Rattus rattus,* *R. norvegicus*	Worldwide	HFRS/moderate	
Arvicoline associated				
Bloodland Lake	*Microtus ochrogaster*	North America	Not recorded	
Puumala	*Clethrionomys glareolus*	Europe	HFRS/mild	Major cause of "nephropathia endemica"
Prospect Hill	*Microtus pennsylvanus*	Eastern United States	Not recorded	
Khabarovsk	*Microtus fortis*	Russia	Not recorded	
Topografov	*Lemmus sibiricus*	Northern Europe	Not recorded	
Tula	*Microtus arvalis*	Europe	Not recorded	
Isla Vista	*Microtus californicus*	Oregon, California, Baja California (Mexico)	Not recorded	
Sigmodontine associated				
Sin Nombre[a]	*Peromyscus maniculatus*	North America	HPS/severe	Causative virus of Four Corners outbreak
New York[b]	*Peromyscus leucopus*	Eastern United States	HPS	
El Moro Canyon	*Reithrodontomys megalotis*	United States, Mexico	Not recorded	
Bayou	*Oryzomys palustris*	SE United States	HPS	
Black Creek Canal	*Sigmodon hispidus*[c]	SE United States	HPS	
Andes[d]	*Oligoryzomys logicaudatus*	Argentina, Chile	HPS/severe	Also renal involvement
Laguna Negra	*Calomys laucha*[c]	Bolivia, Paraguay	HPS	
Rio Mamore	*Oligoryzomys microtis*	Bolivia	Not recorded	
Rio segundo	*Reithrodontomys mexicanus*	Costa Rica	Not recorded	
Other				
Thottapalayam	*Suncus murinus*	India	Not recorded	

[a]Literally "Without name", reflecting the difficulty in naming this virus after the locality in which it was first discovered.

[b]Originally named "Shelter Island" but was renamed after local community objections.

[c]Also reservoirs for arenaviruses.

[d]Variants include: Bermejo, Hu39694, Lechiguanas, Oran and Pergamino viruses.

suspensions of both ticks and tissue samples proved positive in human volunteers. In 1969, Simpson and colleagues demonstrated that the agent of Crimean haemorrhagic fever was identical to a virus isolated in 1956 in the then Congo (now Democratic Republic of Congo). This isolate came from a febrile child in Stanleyville (now Kisango). In recognition of its Eastern European and African distribution the virus is by convention referred to by both geographical names.

Over the last four decades, epidemics due to Crimean-Congo haemorrhagic fever virus have been recognised throughout Europe and many Asian countries. Many of these outbreaks have been nosocomial in origin or the result of a sudden upsurge in human exposure to ticks linked to major land reclamation and resettlement schemes, particularly in the former Soviet Asian republics.

The disease is much less common on the African continent, with only a handful of cases reported each year. Nevertheless, sporadic cases can occur over a wide geographical area, for example several cases of severe disease have been seen in West Africa. In recent years, Crimean-Congo haemorrhagic fever has been diagnosed most frequently in South Africa and Bulgaria—this may reflect more an awareness among clinicians than a circumscribed geographical restriction of the endemic areas. The last major outbreak in the former Soviet republics involved 90 patients in Khazakstan in 1990. However, there has since been a decline in the number of reported cases from this region of the world, possibly due to the rapid change of agricultural practice away from smallholdings to intensive systems of livestock husbandry. This is often coupled with a sharp decline in the natural hosts for the tick vectors, a process accelerated by hunting.

Despite the limited number of cases each year, seroprevalence studies in animals and humans continue to show that the virus is more widespread than the extent of reported cases perhaps suggests. The prevalence of viral antibodies among rural populations rarely exceeds 2%, although 20% has been recorded in Senegal amongst nomadic shepherds. All data point to a significant under-reporting of the disease, although the use of transmission to humans is probably low (Swanepoel, 2000). Most recently, military operations in Afghanistan have revealed Crimean-Congo haemorrhagic fever virus activity along the border regions with Iran to the west and Pakistan to the south east.

Human infections

Crimean-Congo haemorrhagic fever virus causes severe human illness but is not cytopathic for infected cells. Of all the viral haemorrhagic fevers this infection is associated with the most extensive haemorrhagic manifestations, frequently associated with large ecchymoses (Fig. 2). The incubation period after exposure to infected blood is in the order of 5–6 days. This is considerably shorter at 1–3 days if the infection is acquired from an infected tick. The disease has a sudden onset, with symptoms including fever, a severe headache, dizziness, neck pain, photophobia, malaise and myalgia with intense backache or leg pain. Nausea, vomiting and a sore throat are common, with some patients experiencing abdominal pain and diarrhoea.

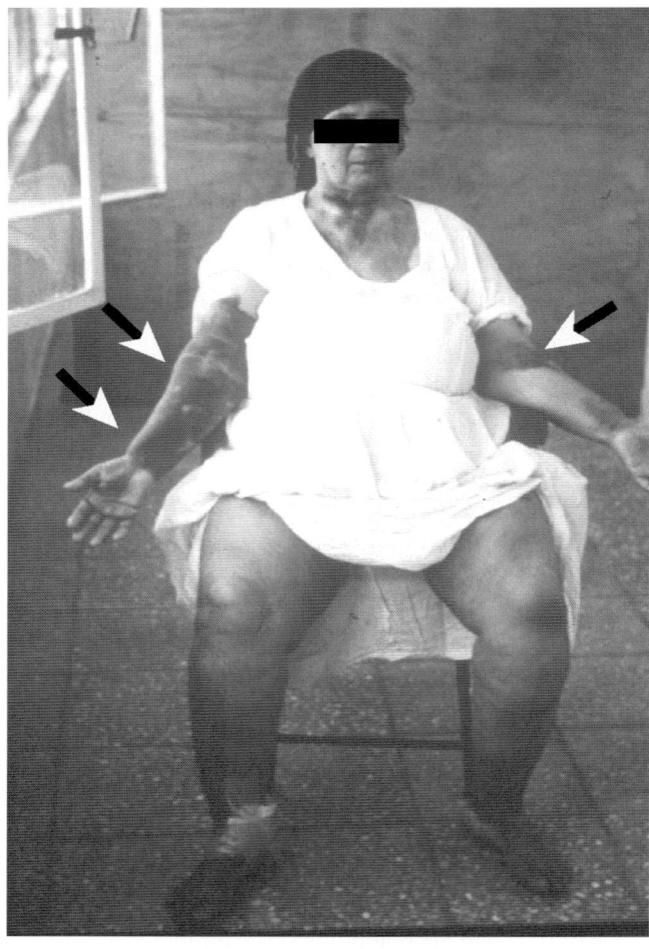

Fig. 2 Patient with acute Congo-Crimean haemorrhagic fever. Note extensive ecchymoses on both forelimbs (courtesy of Professor D.I.H. Simpson).

During the early acute phase, patients undergo abrupt changes of mood accompanied by confusion, lassitude and depression. Signs of liver involvement become apparent by the second to fourth day, with hepatomegaly and abdominal tenderness localised in the upper right quadrant. Tachycardia is frequent and patients are often hypotensive. Other clinical signs include lymphadenopathy and enanthema, and petechiae in the oropharynx.

As the disease progresses a petechial rash develops on the trunk and limbs. This may be followed by extensive bruising and ecchymoses. The development of a haemorrhage may only be apparent from excessive bleeding at venipuncture sites, but epistaxis, haematemesis, haematuria, melaena and generalised bleeding of the gums and orifices often commences by day 5. In severe cases, patients begin to succumb to a generalised failure of the liver, kidneys and lungs, becoming drowsy or comatose. Jaundice is apparent and death generally occurs by the end of the second week.

Diagnosis

Crimean-Congo haemorrhagic fever virus can be isolated from the blood and biopsy material using tissue culture, including Vero, CER and BHK-21 cells. Replication of virus can be detected within 1–5 days post-inoculation using immunofluorescence, but the method is relatively insensitive with virus found only in the blood of severely ill patients during the first 5 days. More sensitive is the intracerebral inoculation of suckling mice, allowing virus detection for a much longer period of up to 2 weeks after onset.

Both virus-specific IgG and IgM antibodies can be detected from the end of the first week of the acute phase in those patients with a good prognosis, and by day 9 all patients in this group show evidence of an antibody response. Recent or ongoing infection is confirmed by either demonstrating a four-fold rise or more in antibody titre or the presence of virus-specific IgM in a single sample. ELISA is the method of choice for antibody detection. IgG antibodies can be detected for at least 5 years after recovery. How long protective immunity lasts is unclear, however. In sharp contrast, antibodies are not found in the blood of severely ill patients with a poor prognosis, diagnosis in these instances being entirely dependent on virus isolation.

Crimean-Congo haemorrhagic fever virus infection needs to be distinguished from other haemorrhagic fevers, and febrile illnesses due to other zoonoses, such as Q fever and brucellosis, that can be acquired from infected animals and animal tissues. In particular, bacterial septicaemias may present with a similar symptomology to Crimean-Congo haemorrhagic fever.

Pathology

Abnormalities are related to the severity of the infection. These include leucopenia or leukocytosis, elevated liver enzymes (AST and ALT), prolonged thrombin and activated partial prothrombin times and elevated levels of fibrin degradation products. Bilirubin, creatinine and urea are also raised in the second week of the acute phase accompanied by a decline in serum protein levels, all indicating a progressive loss of liver function. Histochemical and *in situ* hybridisation shows involvement of both hepatocytes and endothelial cells (Burt et al., 1997).

Histopathological examination of the liver reveals a lack of an inflammatory infiltrate, suggesting that the necrosis in hepatocytes is the direct consequence of virus replication. Necrosis ranges from spotty necrosis in the mid-zonal regions to massive necrosis involving over 75% of the hepatocytes. Lesions in other organs include haemorrhage, congestion and necrosis in the kidneys, CNS and adrenals, accompanied by a general depletion of the lymphoid system. Fibrin deposits may be seen within the blood vessels of these organs.

Treatment and control

The control of Crimean-Congo haemorrhagic fever virus among livestock through the use of acaricides is impractical, especially where arid conditions promote intense animal husbandry. Effective barrier clothing is a must, both for animal handlers and veterinarians, as is the avoidance of blood splashes onto bare skin or into the eyes. Ticks carried on human clothing can be dealt with by use of any number of pyrethroid compounds.

Attempts to produce a vaccine against Crimean-Congo haemorrhagic fever virus have been confined to Eastern Europe and the former Soviet Union. Several human trials were conducted some 20 years ago but the results of these were not conclusive and not widely disseminated. Given the sporadic nature of Crimean-Congo haemorrhagic fever and the relatively small numbers of persons at risk, it is highly unlikely that a vaccine for human use will be forthcoming in the foreseeable future.

Rift Valley fever

Rift Valley fever was named as a result of its first being discovered in the Rift Valley of East Africa. Spread by arthropod vectors, several major epidemics have occurred at irregular intervals, largely as a result of climatic changes and man-generated alterations to irrigation systems along the Nile, particularly in upper Egypt. A member of the *Phlebovirus* genus, Rift Valley fever virus has amongst all of the bunyaviruses the greatest potential to cause serious economic loss to the livestock industry should it spread to Europe and North America. Forewarnings of this risk are the recent outbreaks in the Horn of Africa and on the Arabian Peninsula. Additionally, large epidemics in African populations have also illustrated that Rift Valley fever virus represents a real cause for concern should this virus be introduced by accident or by design into these areas where mosquito competence would ensure its survival, posing a threat among humans and animals alike.

The genus *Phlebovirus* takes its name after the phlebotomous vector of Sandfly fever, a disease known for over two centuries (now known, in fact, to be two distinct viruses: Sandfly Fever Naples and Sandfly Fever Sicilian). Zinga virus, originally isolated in the Central African Republic in 1969, and Lunyo virus, isolated in Uganda in 1969, are both now known to be strains of Rift Valley fever virus.

Rift Valley fever virus is an acute disease of domestic ruminants of East Africa and Madagascar transmitted by mosquitoes of the *Aedes* and *Culex* families. After having been restricted to sub-Saharan Africa, Rift Valley fever virus spread suddenly northward to Egypt in 1977, an event that dramatically showed how a zoonosis can, without warning, become a serious threat to both human and animal health. There have since been further smaller, but continuing outbreaks in Egypt and a much larger outbreak in Mauritania in 1987. In 1998 Rift Valley fever caused an extensive outbreak in Kenya and

Somalia following abnormal rainfall that year. Over the past 25 years, Rift Valley fever has continued to expand in geographical distribution and in the last decade has gained a foothold on the Arabian Peninsula.

Many different mosquito vectors have the capacity to carry and amplify Rift Valley fever virus and the introduction of intensive farming of livestock farming increases the potential risk of further outbreaks. Of all the bunyaviruses capable of crippling the public infrastructure for dealing with infectious disease, Rift Valley fever virus ranks among the greatest of risks (see Comment and perspectives for further discussion).

Morphology and structure

Virus particles are spherical, approximately 100 nm in diameter, with a lipid envelope through which project virus-encoded glycoproteins. The surface morphology of RVF virus is distinct, showing small round subunits with a central core (Fig. 3).

Genetic properties and replication

The S RNA segment has an ambisense coding strategy for the expression of the nucleo-capsid (N) protein and a non-structural protein (NSs). The N gene is first transcribed by the viral RNA polymerase to generate sub-genomic virus complementary sense mRNA. The NSs protein is expressed by the generation of a sub-genomic virus sense mRNA that is transcribed by the viral RNA polymerase from a full-length antigenome S RNA template (Fig. 1). The NSs protein is transported to the nucleus immediately after synthesis, suggesting a regulatory function at the level of host RNA synthesis. The NSs protein accumulates and produces the intra-nuclear filamentous forms that are a histopathological feature of infected cells and tissues (Yadani et al., 1999). Here NSs

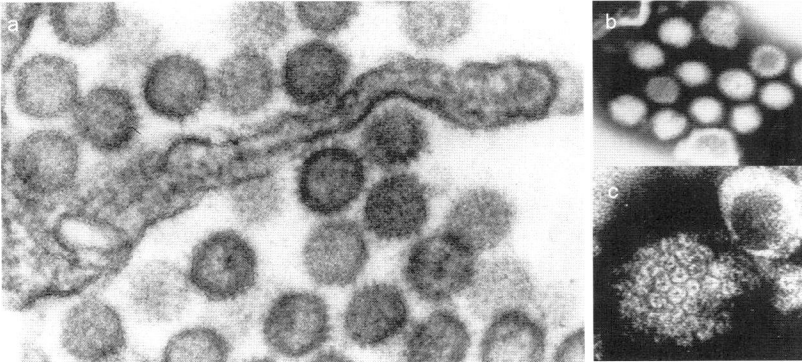

Fig. 3 Electron microscopy of CCHF virus budding from Vero cell cultures (a), negative staining electron microscopy of Rift Valley fever virus particles (b) and extracellular CCHF virus particle showing detail of surface structures (c) (courtesy of Dr D.S. Ellis).

interacts with the host transcription factor TFIIH, leading to a precipitate decline in cellular RNA synthesis, one immediate consequence likely being a cessation in interferon synthesis in response to virus infection (Le May et al., 2004).

The envelope glycoproteins Gn and Gc bear the ligands for the cellular receptors and antibody to these confers immunity. As is characteristic of all bunyaviruses, nascent virions mature principally at the Golgi, through which new particles bud into vacuoles before being transported to the cell surface. There is some evidence of budding directly at the plasma membrane.

Background and epidemiology

Rift Valley fever first came to prominence in Kenya in 1931 when an outbreak occurred in sheep and man, although it is likely however, that cases were recorded as long ago as 1912. It was found that the infection could be transmitted by filtrates of blood and liver homogenate to unexposed sheep.

It has been assumed that such epidemics may have been triggered by the importation from Europe and elsewhere of sheep and other livestock that were more susceptible to infection than the indigenous fauna of the time. Coupled with the introduction of intensive agricultural methods the chances of Rift Valley fever becoming established and broadening its host range were magnified considerably.

Between epidemics the virus is maintained in endemic areas by *Aedes* species, as was eloquently shown in the early 1980s by Linthicum et al. (1985) when virus was successfully isolated from *Aedes macintoshi* from a ranch in Kenya. Other *Aedes* species also can play a role in maintaining the virus in the environment, such as *A. dentatus*, *A. unidentatus* and *A. juppi*. *A. macintoshi* is the most important of these, however, as the virus can also be maintained in this species by transovarial passage. Epidemics occur as a result of heavy rainfall when there is a rapid upsurge in mosquito numbers in those areas already populated by infected mosquitoes. The numbers of infected vectors multiplies dramatically, thus escalating the risk of animals acquiring the infection. Further amplification of the disease occurs as a consequence of virus acquisition by other *Aedes* as well as *Culex* species not involved in virus maintenance during the drier, inter-epidemic periods.

Of all the haemorrhagic fevers, Rift Valley fever seems the most linked to climatic change. There have been moves to introduce predictive mechanisms of epidemics in sub-Saharan Africa using meteorological data and remote sensing by satellite (Linthicum et al., 1999). Above average rainfall favours the breeding of the mosquito vectors. In Southern and East Africa sheep rearing is carried out on the high plateaus and uplands. During times of above average rainfall—usually every 10–15 years—surface water collects in shallow depressions (pans) or in low-lying grassy areas (dambos) and these make excellent breeding grounds for *Aedes* mosquitoes. Surveillance studies in Zimbabwe have shown that between epidemics there is a continuing level of virus activity in both mosquitoes and animals, albeit at a much reduced level. There is hence no need after heavy rainfall for incursions from adjacent endemic areas for epidemics to occur. Satellite images and aerial photography show an almost complete concordance between endemic zones and the accumulation of surface water. Linthicum et al. (1985) artificially flooded a dambo of some 1800 m^2 and as a result recovered nearly a million adult mosquitoes belonging to species known to carry Rift Valley fever virus. Virus was recovered from both male and female insects reared in the laboratory from larvae recovered from naturally and artificially flooded dambos.

The spread of Rift Valley fever virus up the Nile Valley of East Africa into Egypt in 1977 sparked off the worst epidemic in humans recorded to date. The effect on local livestock was devastating with an estimated 25–50% of all sheep and cattle in the region infected. There was extensive spread to humans between September and December of that year, with a probable 200,000 infections and over 600 deaths. In some areas, human infections exceeded 35%. This outbreak coincided with major changes in irrigation channels as a result of the building of the Aswan dam on the Upper Nile. The major vector seems to have been *Culex pipiens*. Rift Valley fever returned to Egypt in 1993 and outbreaks have continued to occur since. The virus has also spread to Madagascar, and north into the Horn of Africa, largely as a result of abnormal rainfall resulting from climatic conditions influenced by the El Niño Southern Oscillation.

Rift Valley fever in livestock

RVF is primarily a veterinary public health problem on the African continent. Newborn lambs and kid goats are the most susceptible agricultural livestock. It is estimated that there are at any one time over 1200 million sheep and goats being husbanded worldwide, a high proportion of these in Africa. The importance of these species to the economy of sub-Saharan Africa cannot be overestimated. In the 1997 outbreak in Kenya and Somalia, losses to farmers and nomads amounted to over 70% of livestock with dire consequences for their brittle economies.

The short incubation period of around 24 h is followed by a marked fever and the animals quickly become inappetent and listless accompanied by hypernoea. The disease has a short progression and over 90% of lambs and kids succumb by 3 days after exposure. Lambs and kids older than 2 weeks are far less susceptible, most developing an acute disease from which 40–90% recover. During the acute phase there are signs of haemorrhage with malaena and a bloody nasal discharge, occasionally accompanied by symptoms of liver involvement. It is possible that a proportion of infections is unapparent, and therefore goes unnoticed by herdsmen and farmers. Abortion is thus the first indication of the disease among flocks and herds. Pregnant ewes may abort at any time during gestation. Abortion rates vary, with figures in the literature from 40 to 100%.

Outbreaks of Rift Valley fever are normally preceded by periods of heavy rainfall. Other infections can occur simultaneously with the re-emergence of Rift Valley fever and thus complicate a diagnosis. Wesselbron disease in particular can cause mortality in young livestock, although at rates lower than those normally associated with Rift Valley fever. Adult animals are also much less susceptible to Wesselbron's disease. Nairobi sheep disease also causes hepatitis, abortion and mortality in sheep and goats. Non-viral causes of hepatitis involvement and haemorrhage include the bacterial septicaemias, such as salmonellosis, pasteurellosis and anthrax, as well as contagious pustular dermatitis, bluetongue, foot rot and non-specific pneumonia. The movement of livestock away from temporary flooding to higher ground may compound the difficulties by exposing animals to foot and mouth virus and morbillivirus infections.

The disease in cattle appears more benign, with an attendant risk that infection of cattle may go unnoticed. As with sheep and goats, it is newborn calves that are most at risk, developing clinical signs very similar to those seen in ovines. The acute disease in cattle, both among calves and adults, tends to be more prolonged, ranging from 8 to 20 days, respectively.

The level of virus in infected animals is high, with viraemia in excess of 10^{10} LD_{50} infectious doses for mice being recorded for isolates from lambs, 10^8 in the blood of kids and 10^7 in calves (Swanepoel, 2000). Such titres imply that RVF virus has a particularly high capacity for replication in animals yet to develop a functioning immune system. Such high viraemias also present the maximum opportunity for fresh cycles of vector-mediated transmission.

Other species are susceptible, such as the African buffalo and camels. Although transient fever and a viraemia are likely, these species do not appear to be major hosts. Horses develop only a low-grade viraemia when experimentally infected and pigs and dogs can only support sub-clinical infections. Birds appear to be totally resistant to infection.

Active surveillance coupled with regular monitoring of rainfall patterns are key to predicting the emergence of fresh outbreaks. The benefits of such an approach are amply illustrated by the 1997 outbreak in north-eastern Kenya and western Somalia. This followed an abnormal period of rainfall, between 60 and 100 times that is normally experienced in this region each year. The combined efforts of local health authorities and local representatives of the World Health Organisation did much to stem this outbreak. Around 370 human deaths due to a haemorrhagic condition had been reported, mainly in the Garissa region of Kenya bordering Somalia. Evidence of Rift Valley fever was quickly found by rapid screening of samples for IgM antibodies, virus isolation, immunohistochemistry and confirmatory PCR tests. The surprise was that only 23% of cases were directly attributable to Rift Valley fever virus. Notwithstanding this low percentage, a detailed cross-sectional survey showed that at least 27,500 infections had occurred, by far the largest outbreak of Rift Valley fever recorded in sub-Saharan Africa for twenty years. This number is doubled if the number of IgG positive sera is taken into account, meaning that some 23% of the total human population had been exposed. Risk factors included exposure to livestock, contact with animal blood and tissues, amniotic fluid or with milk but excluding its consumption.

The puzzle of this outbreak was the cause of the severe disease seen in the remaining three quarters of the clinical cases negative for markers of Rift Valley fever virus. The cloning of PCR products revealed a new recombinant virus, one that contained both the L and S RNA segments of bunyamwera virus (a member of the *Bunyavirus* genus) and a unique M RNA segment. This is surprising, as bunyamwera virus is not normally associated with human infections and certainly not ranked as among the agents causing haemorrhagic fevers. The M segment produced a further surprise with the nucleotide sequence showing a somewhat less than 80% identity to Cache Valley virus, another member of the bunyavirus family found in North America. This new agent, dubbed Garissa virus, represented a reassortment virus that presumably has arisen as a result of dual infection with bunyamwera and some other hitherto identified agent distantly related to Cache Valley virus (Bowen et al., 2001). The result has been the emergence of a recombinant virus with substantial virulence for humans. It was clear during the Garissa outbreak that infection due to the new recombinant virus occurred independently of Rift Valley fever infection.

Human infections

The most extensively documented human outbreak occurred in 1977 in and around Cairo, an area ideal for the breeding of carrier mosquitoes (Meegan, 1979) (Fig. 4).

Of all the viral haemorrhagic fevers, Rift Valley fever virus has the most variable clinical presentation. After an incubation period of 2–6 days Rift Valley fever in humans has a sudden onset characterised by fever and rigor. The febrile period persists for 2–3 days, the fever is frequently biphasic, and accompanied by headache, muscle and joint pains, and photophobia. Virus can be recovered from the blood with a titre in excess of 10^8 ID_{50} per ml, as measured by inoculation of suckling mice. Despite the high virus titre in blood, there are no substantive reports of person-to-person transmission, either directly or via arthropods. Nausea and vomiting accompanied by abdominal pain are sometimes recorded. In most patients, convalescence quickly follows with recovery by the end of the second week of illness. There are no adverse sequelae in benign cases, save in instances where there is an ocular involvement. This may lead to a temporary impairment of vision that persists well into convalescence. The ocular lesion is one of a focal retinal ischemia

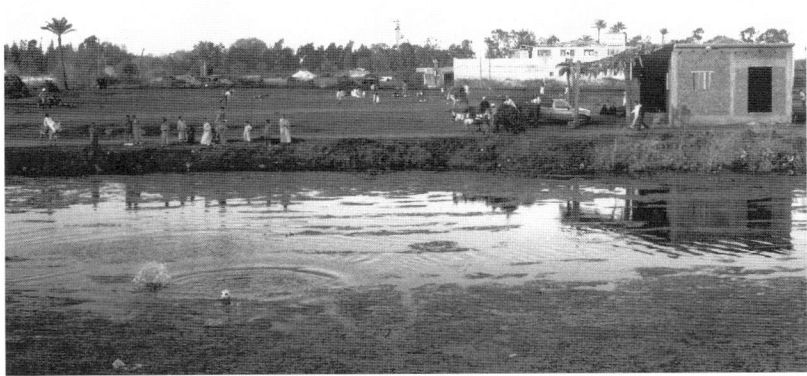

Fig. 4 Irrigation canals, Cairo, Egypt. Expansive areas of still water encourage breeding of *Culex* and other mosquito species capable of transmitting Rift Valley fever (photograph by the author).

resulting from minute thrombi obstructing the ocular arterioles of the retina in the macular and paramacular regions (Fig. 5). In severe cases, this can cause retinal detachment and an exudate sufficient to result in a loss of optical transparency (Siam et al., 1980). Although the lesions eventually resolved, around half of such cases in the Egyptian outbreak led to a permanent loss of visual acuity.

It is thought that extensive involvement of the liver can result in the haemorrhagic form of severe disease. The first signs of haemorrhage appear during the acute phase, most notably by the appearance of petechiae. These can progress quickly into purpura and extensive ecchymoses. Bleeding occurs at venipuncture sites, at the gingival crevice and at other sites including the gastrointestinal tract. The haemorrhagic form is accompanied by an intense jaundice, renal failure and cardiopulmonary arrest. Among those survivors, recovery is prolonged but eventually complete. An encephalitis is occasionally seen accompanying haemorrhagic manifestations and in more moderate cases. In the latter, the onset of encephalitis can occur at any time and as late as 3 weeks into convalescence. Encephalitic patients may well be left with long-term sequelae, for example hemiparesis.

Various sources estimate the case fatality rate in humans is less than 1%. The Egyptian outbreak of 1977 accounted for nearly 600 deaths among 200,000 recorded

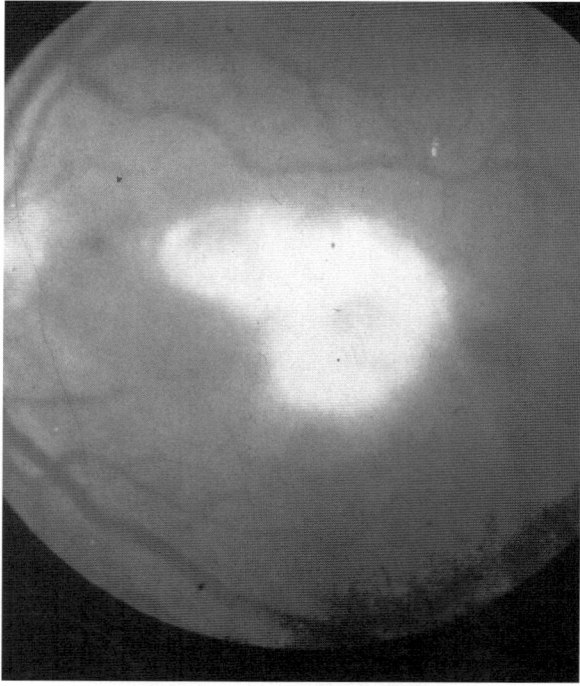

Fig. 5 Retinopathy in a case of Human Rift Valley fever during the 1977 outbreak (photograph courtesy of Professor D.I.H. Simpson).

cases, although this number almost certainly is a considerable underestimate. Seroprevalence studies within the affect area suggest as many as 30% of the local population may have been exposed to the virus.

As hepatitis is invariably present the disease on presentation needs to be clearly distinguished from viral hepatitis, especially hepatitis A, which is frequently present in endemic areas. Rift Valley fever also needs to be distinguished from Q fever and brucellosis, as well as other causes of viral haemorrhagic disease.

Diagnosis

A PCR method for the detection of Rift Valley fever virus RNA in mosquitoes has been developed by Ibrahim et al. (1997). Using primers flanking a conserved 551 bp portion of the Gn glycoprotein gene on the M RNA segment, these workers were able to detect a single infected mosquito in a pool of 25–50 insects. The sensitivity of this assay is largely dependent upon the method of RNA extraction, however, as Trizol extraction leaves residues capable of interfering with the polymerase reaction. Thus, insect samples need to be further extracted with phenol–chloroform to ensure the removal of such inhibitors.

Viral antigen can be detected in the blood using standard serological assays, e.g. ELISA. Viraemia lasts up to 7 days after onset, and the virus can easily be isolated in cell cultures readily available in most routine clinical virology laboratories. Confirmation of virus growth is best undertaken by immunofluorescent staining of the infected cell cultures. Mice are the most sensitive species for virus isolation, although there are differences in murine susceptibility according to mouse haplotype.

As with other acute viral infections, a four-fold rise in total antibody titre in paired samples or the presence of IgM antibodies in a single sample is indicative of recent or ongoing virus infection.

Pathology

Histopathological examination of the liver is useful for the diagnosis of disease in both humans and animals. Lesions vary in severity from necrotic foci containing clusters of hepatocytes with acidophilic cytoplasms and pyknotic nuclei to massive necrosis leaving only narrow areas of intact hepatocytes around the portal tracts. The acidophilic cytoplasmic bodies resemble the Councilman bodies more generally associated with yellow fever (see Flaviviruses and Fig. 5). Rod shaped or round eosinophilic intranuclear inclusions are evident in the nuclei.

Considerable progress has been made in unravelling the early stages of the disease process. There appears to be an age-dependent susceptibility to infection. Parallel studies with the bunyavirus La Crosse virus have shown that newborn mice develop high tires of viraemia and death quickly ensues. In contrast, older animals are able to contain the infection, thus the chance of survival rises rapidly with age. This age-dependent response to infection suggests that innate immunity, not fully developed in newborns, plays a key role in recovery from infection. Type 1 interferons are important mediators of innate immunity and the addition of IFN-α to cell cultures inhibits Rift Valley fever virus replication. This effect is mediated by the induction of Mx proteins (large GTPases) which sequester viral N protein, thereby depleting the viral RNA synthesis mechanism of an essential factor for RNA polymerase activity (Kochs, 2002). This is consistent with the observation that mice deficient in Mx protein are highly sensitive to La Crosse virus, whereas wild type mice only succumb when infected at or shortly after birth (Hefti et al., 1999).

Rift Valley fever virus is directly cytolytic for a variety of endothelial cells in culture. Little is known as to the detailed pathogenesis of Rift Valley fever virus save what has been learnt from experimental infection of monkeys. Again alpha interferon (IFN-α) seems to have a pivotal role: a strong IFN-α response within 6–12 h of exposure signals the development of a mild disease. The longer the delay in IFN-α production, the greater the disease severity becomes and the poorer the prognosis. The severe disease is manifested by extensive disruption of the haemopoietic system, including disseminated intravascular coagulation (DIC), haemolytic anaemia and intravascular deposition of fibrin thrombi. The delay in the interferon response probably increases the extent to which vascular epithelium becomes infected and the anti-thrombotic lining of the capillaries becomes damaged by virus replication, particularly in the kidneys.

Animal models

The susceptibility of mice has been used as a model of Rift Valley fever virus pathogenesis. Despite being carried out over 45 years ago, the work of Cedric Mims remains seminal in understanding the pathogenesis of Rift Valley fever virus, and indeed ranks among the earliest attempts to understand the process whereby viruses disseminate and cause abnormal functions in target organs.[1] Mims showed that virus travelled from the periphery to the draining lymph nodes where primary replication takes place, probably in lymphatic macrophages. The liver then becomes rapidly infected and this organ is the most likely source of the resulting high titre viraemia during the acute phase. The blood–brain barrier can be breached, with a meningo-encephalitis and a retinitis seen 2–3 weeks after infection, although these responses are the consequences of an inflammatory response. Different strains of rat show markedly different responses to an individual virus isolate. Some rat strains are resistant and quickly seroconvert, others develop a fatal fulminant hepatitis and some an encephalitis. Interestingly, those rat strains resistant to infection appear to have a mechanism that restricts virus replication in the liver (Anderson et al., 1987).

Treatment

Patients are provided supportive therapy including the replacement of blood and coagulation factors. It is known that ribavirin will inhibit Rift Valley fever virus

---

[1] For a general introduction to viral pathogenesis, the reader is strongly recommended *Mim's Pathogenesis of Infectious Diseases (5th edn.)* by C.A. Mims, A. Nash and J. Stephen, Academic Press, 2000, ISBN 0124 982 646.

replication in cell culture, but there are no data regarding its effectiveness in the clinical treatment of Rift Valley fever.

IFN-α therapy is a possibility for treatment. The hepatitis suggests the liver is a major site of virus replication, and as with hepatitis B treatment of patients with IFN-α may serve to interfere with host support of the replication process. Work in animal models has shown that immune plasma can be effective, but this has not been attempted in clinical practice.

Vaccination against RVF

Attempts to produce effective vaccines began in the 1930s. Both chemically-inactivated vaccines and chemically-attenuated vaccines have been produced for veterinary use, whereas only inactivated vaccines have been developed for humans.

Veterinary vaccines

Livestock vaccination can protect against arthropod transmission and therefore interrupt amplification of the virus and spread to humans. Coupled with surveillance of vegetation and rainfall, control of human disease is possible without necessarily introducing widespread vaccination among human populations. In any event, epizootics can occur outside of these regions traditionally regarded as endemic for Rift Valley fever. Unfortunately, livestock vaccines have a pedigree of being excessively reactogenic, and this coupled with reluctance on the part of owners to use vaccines outside of epidemic periods means vaccine coverage in East Africa is almost certainly below the level that would effectively guard against repeated outbreaks.

The thrust of projects designed to develop attenuated vaccines has been to moderate the pantropic nature of Rift Valley fever virus—over the years there have been many such attempts to achieve this, primarily using consecutive passages in mice. Such strains are not entirely attenuated, however, in that they remain neurotropic. As early as 1936 a neurotropic strain passaged previously a total of 92 times in mouse brain was used during the 1936–1937 outbreak in Kenya. This crude vaccine was effective in ewes and lambs over 6 months old, but caused fatal encephalitis in newborns and abortions in pregnant ewes.

Two veterinary vaccines are available for use in farm animals. The first is a live attenuated product consisting of the Smithburn strain of Rift Valley fever virus that is particularly recommended for non-pregnant sheep. This strain was isolated from mosquitoes in Uganda in 1944 and passaged intracerebrally in adult mice before being passaged in Foetal Rhesus Lung (FRhL) cell cultures in order to produce a seed lot.

Smithburn reported in 1949 that intraperitoneal inoculation of sheep with mouse brain virus by the 83–85 passage level were fully protected against challenge with pantropic virus. Significantly, Smithburn showed that maternal immunity could be transferred to lambs, an important finding: it appears with all bunyaviruses that antibody is sufficient to confer protection. Despite a number of attempts to further attenuate the Smithburn strain by a variety of means, the original 102nd passage provided the basis for further vaccine development. Historically, live attenuated vaccines have found considerable use: for example, over 18 million doses were used to contain the 1975 epidemic in South Africa.

The Smithburn attenuated vaccine induces lifelong protection on sheep and goats if given between 6 and 12 months of age. The problem is that this vaccine is teratogenic: pregnant ewes inoculated 5–10 weeks after gestation with this vaccine can result in a range of foetal abnormalities in around 2% of animals. These abnormalities are particularly focused on the central nervous system (Barnard and Botha, 1977). Immunisation earlier in pregnancy may lead to loss of the conceptus which may go unnoticed, and inoculation later than 10 weeks can induce abortion of the foetus. Coupled with the high risk of reversion and possible recombination with co-circulating wild type strains, this vaccine is of very limited use between epidemics. In addition, it is of limited use in cattle as the process of attenuation appears to have resulted in reduced immunogenicity for the bovine immune system.

There have been other attempts at producing a live attenuated vaccine for veterinary use. One such programme focused on use of virus isolated from a patient confined to the Zanzig Hospital during the 1977 Egyptian outbreak. This ZH-548 strain was derived by passage twice in suckling mice, once in FRhL cells, and then 12 times in MRC-5 cells in the presence of 200 μg/ml of 5-fluorouracil to encourage mutagenesis of the viral genome. A seed lot was then prepared by a further passage of in MRC-5 cells in the absence of 5-fluorouracil. This vaccine was fully attenuated for mice and farm animals with little sign of reversion. Trials demonstrated that this vaccine possesses good immunogenicity for farm animals with no evidence of spread to handlers and stockmen.

The second vaccine is a chemically inactivated product specifically designed for use in cattle. A wild type isolate was adapted in 1971 for growth in FRhL cell cultures. The cell-grown virus is harvested 4 days after infection at the point when the virus-induced cytopathogenicity results in destruction of the cell monolayer. Apart from removal of cell debris, the vaccine is not purified prior to inactivation with formalin using a standard inactivation protocol (Swanepoel, 2000).

Barnard and Botha (1977) reported alternative ways of preparing an inactivated veterinary vaccine that alleviated the abortigenic properties, is immunogenic for cattle, and minimised the risk of transmission to animal handlers. Experimentally such a candidate vaccine was less than ideal: although immunised sheep did not develop clinical disease in challenge with wild type virus, a viraemia was detected in up to 40% of the challenged animals. Nevertheless, it proved effective in controlling the disease during an outbreak. Generally there have been a number of attempts to increase the immunogenicity of inactivated vaccines by use of lipid adjuvants and poly(ICLC) (Barnard, 1979; Harrington et al., 1980; Reynolds et al., 1980).

Investigators in the United States responded to the Egyptian outbreak of 1977 with an evaluation of the U.S. human candidate NDBK-103 product (see below) as a possible animal vaccine. Trials in sheep and cattle met with varying degrees of success (Yedloutschnig et al., 1979; Harrington et al., 1980). As could have been expected from an inactivated vaccine, single doses were largely ineffective in preventing infection on challenge with ZH-501, a well-characterised Egyptian human isolate.

Human vaccines

The use of inactivated human vaccines was first pioneered in 1935 using virus isolated from mice. A further 30 years were to elapse before renewed efforts were made using the Entebbe strain, propagated in monkey cell cultures. All of 107 volunteers aged between 19 and 24 developed antibody titres in the range of 48–436, in excess of the 1:40 titre of neutralising antibodies regarded as the minimum for protection. However, as may be expected with an inactivated vaccine, booster doses were required at 6 months: a prompt anamnestic response was observed, with the extent of the secondary response dependent upon the titre of antibodies at the end of primary immunisation (Kark et al., 1985).

The vaccine, labelled as NDBK-103, was subsequently used as a prophylactic immunogen in Swedish troops deployed in the Sinai as part of a UN force stationed there in 1979. Side effects were limited to individual cases of herpes zoster reactivation, cardiac arrhythmia and a presumptive case of Guillaime-Barre syndrome. This vaccine was further refined by passage in FRL cells, the resulting product identified by the term TSI-GSD-200. The resulting vaccine was subsequently proved to be safe and immunogenic in a trial of over a 1000 volunteers (Eddy and Peters, 1980) and has been used successfully to prevent laboratory outbreaks (Kark et al., 1982).

Laboratory infections with Rift Valley fever have been common and thus there have been determined efforts to develop vaccines suitable for human use. The United States Department of Defense has developed several candidate vaccines at various times. The first of these, an attenuated vaccine (MP-12) developed in the 1980s by growth in the presence of 5-fluorouracil (Caplen et al., 1985), successfully completed a phase I safety trial in over 60 healthy volunteers. The MP-12 vaccine has also been extensively evaluated in domestic livestock and again found to be safe, particularly in pregnant ewes (Morrill et al., 1987, 1991). As part of these studies, it was also shown that female *Culex pipiens* mosquitoes fed on immunised animals failed to transmit Rift Valley fever virus to hamsters, an important confirmation not only of vaccine efficiency in interrupting the insect animal transmission cycle but again in showing the value of neutralising antibodies for protection.

A more modern inactivated product based on the TSI-GSD-200 strain has been developed by American investigators. This is an inactivated preparation of virus grown in cell cultures after plaque cloning in a line of diploid foetal rhesus monkey lung cells. This vaccine is safe and well tolerated in volunteers. The assumption in these trials has been that a neutralising antibody titre of 1:40 or greater equates with a protective antibody response, and over 90% develop antibodies at a level equal or greater than this after completing a course of injections delivered at 0, 7 and 28 days (Pittman et al., 1999). The half-life of these antibodies was such that over half the volunteers remained antibody-positive after 6 years, provided a boost was given at 12 months. Fortunately, there is no evidence of significant variation in the critical domains that react with neutralising antibodies, and thus at present there is every confidence that a single vaccine product will provide laboratory and healthcare workers against Rift Valley fever working with samples from different geographical regions.

Hantaviruses

The genus *Hantavirus* contains an ever-increasing number of agents. These viruses are associated with HFRS in Asia and Europe, or HPS in the Americas. Unlike viruses in other genera of the Bunyaviridae, hantaviruses are not transmitted by arthropods: both rodent and human infections are acquired by the aerosol route or by close contact with contaminated surfaces. Hantaviruses are primarily infections of rodents, with humans acting only as incidental hosts when exposed to rodent excreta. Distributed almost worldwide, endemic regions are found in the Americas, Europe and Asia. Curiously, hantaviruses have not been recorded from Africa. These viruses are also absent from Australia and New Zealand where it is believed the fauna necessary to act as host reservoirs do not exist.

Classification

Over 20 hantaviruses have now been identified (Table 1). Each occupies a unique ecological niche, causing a chronic persistent infection in a specific rodent species or subspecies. These differences have been the subject of extensive phylogenetic analyses. Sequence comparisons show at least 7% difference in amino acid composition of the envelope glycoprotein precursor and nucleocapsid (N) proteins coded by the M RNA segment between hantaviruses infecting different rodent species, with at least a four-fold difference in cross-neutralisation assays. Less exact is the criterion that a hantavirus species can be defined by a lack of reassortment between RNA segments as reassortments can be readily generated in the laboratory. Almost all hantaviruses have taken names from those geographical areas associated with the infected hosts: one (Prospect Hill) was named after the homestead in Maryland, USA from which the infected rodent was trapped.

At least seven hantaviruses have been fully sequenced, including Hantaan, Dobrava, Puumala and Sin Nombre viruses: these account for the vast majority of human infections so far recorded. Importantly, the newer isolates have been identified on the basis of sequence analyses rather than the more conventional approach of virus isolation in cell culture. This is in sharp contrast with the situation within other genera of the family Bunyaviridae where virus isolation has been the norm and there is a paucity of sequence data, particularly amongst viruses not hitherto suspected of causing significant animal or human disease. Thus, although much can be said regard to the individual genetic relationships between the different hantaviruses, it is much more difficult to relate these to antigenic and biological properties.

Sequence analyses reveal hantaviruses are evolving primarily by a process of genetic drift, with a steady accumulation of nucleotide deletions and substitutions, especially in the non-coding regions at either end of the viral RNA segments. There is evidence for reassortment and, importantly, for recombination between homologous regions of two different parental RNA segments, events that seem to play a role in "host-switching" when viruses jump from the otherwise straight confines of a single rodent host (see next section for a fuller discussion). The latter process can confound considerably both comparative genome analyses and studies attempting to link sequence changes with the potential to cause disease in humans.

There has been extensive debate between workers in the field as to just what constitutes a new hantavirus species, especially given the heavy reliance on sequence data *in lieu* of more conventional neutralisation of infectivity assays employing convalescent and hyperimmune antisera. The ICTV report in its 7th Edition has attempted to help define new species by adopting a number of criteria (Table 2). Owing to the tight association between each hantavirus and a single rodent species, the characteristics of an individual isolate may reflect the habitat and behaviour of the host as much as, if not more than, its propensity to cause human disease. That serology has a useful role, however, is admirably shown by work on a virus first found on Saaremaa Island, part of Estonia. Serology showed this new hantavirus was a distinct species rather than a variant of Dobrava virus, as was originally thought (Sjolander et al., 2002). This is consistent with the far less pathogenic nature of Saaremaa virus compared to Dobrava virus, and also the finding that both viruses can co-circulate in their respective hosts within the same locality.

Natural history and the virus–host relationship

Hantaviruses cause zoonotic diseases, primarily associated with the rodent family Muridae. Because of the exquisitely tight relationship between virus and host, with each rodent species being infected with a single virus (Schmaljohn and Hjelle, 1997) outbreaks of human disease are tightly circumscribed by the geographical distribution of the host rodent species.

Hantaviruses show a close relationship with their native rodent hosts. For example, the agent of HFRS is intimately associated with the field rodent *Apodemus agrarius*, the most common field rodent over much of northern and eastern Asia. It readily invades cultivated areas, gardens and barns, with incursions into human dwellings more frequent when rodent numbers increase. There is much heightened interest in this relationship and the causative agents of Hantavirus pulmonary syndrome (HPS), especially since the Four Corners outbreak of HPS in the USA in 1993. One exception to this relationship between rodent and virus seems to be Thottapalyan virus, an agent recovered from the shrew

Table 2

Criteria recommended by the International Committee for the Taxonomy of Viruses (ICTV) in respect to classifying new species of hantaviruses

Criteria
Virus found in a unique ecological niche, i.e. in a distinct primary rodent host species or subspecies
Do not readily form genetic reassortments with other hantavirus species
Exhibit at least 7% difference in amino acid sequence of the complete GPC (glycoprotein precursor) and nucleocapsid (N) protein
Show at least a fourfold difference in two-way cross-neutralisation tests

Suncus murinus. It is unclear whether the latter represents a unique association with an insectivore or a chance isolation: a similar paradox is the isolation in Trinidad of the arenavirus Tacaribe virus from an *Artibeus* fruit bat.

Hantaan virus is the prototype of the genus *Hantavirus*. Dr Ho Wang Lee and his colleagues at the Seoul National University were the first to isolate the causative agent in 1978 from the lungs of a captured *A. agrarius* field vole. This common feral rodent is the major rodent host of the virus now referred to as Hantaan virus after the Hantaan River which flows through the Korean peninsula close to the demilitarised zone.

As is so often the case with zoonotic diseases, changes in local environment and climatic conditions can increase substantially the risk of transmission of hantaviruses to humans. The 1993 hantavirus outbreak on the Colorado Plateau of the USA instigated intensive research into understanding better the fluctuations in rodent populations and identifying risk factors associated with human disease. Simplistically, abnormal weather patterns resulting in increased rainfall led to a dramatic increase in vegetation suitable as food for rodents, with the result that the environment was able to sustain suddenly the rapidly expanding numbers of rodents. Generally as rodent population sizes explode, so the chance of rodents entering peridomestic areas increases. This leads to a rise in the incidence of human illness as individuals have that much greater chance of coming into contact with excreta from persistently infected animals. The chance of virus switching into other rodent species also increases. The geography of the terrain significantly affects virus transmission, with areas representing the greatest risk being mainly at the higher elevations.

Glass et al. (2002) examined in some detail what is termed the "trophic cascade hypothesis", comparing satellite images of vegetation with rodent population numbers in high and low areas of disease prevalence. A significant correlation was found between the numbers of trapped rodents carrying the Sin Nombre virus, human infections and the flora providing food for *Peromyscus* deer mice. During the period 1998–1999 abnormal weather patterns attributable to the El Niño Southern Oscillation and similar to those previously experienced in 1992 occurred once more over the south-western USA. This in turn led to a marked increase in the prevalence of virus infections in high risk areas, with a lag of approximately 1 year between the end of the weather cycle and outbreaks of HPS. Such lag periods are due to virus amplification within the expanded rodent populations, with evidence of infection in 36% or more of adult *P. maniculatus* trapped in high risk areas. This was in sharp contrast to the 8.3% prevalence found in deer mice trapped in areas predicted as representing a much lower risk (Glass et al., 2002). In areas where there is a low risk to humans, rodent populations survive for less than 2 years: these regions only become re-populated once again when rodent colonists overspill from high risk areas at those times when an abundance of food is available. Crucial to these dynamics is the time it takes for hantaviruses to become established. Dependent as Sin Nombre virus is upon horizontal transmission, it is likely that colonies of deer mice do not survive long enough for the virus to become established, and as a consequence the risk to human communities is considerably reduced compared to what it might be if horizontal transmission was a regular occurrence.

Switching to a new rodent species can have a profound effect on the evolution of hantaviruses. Adaptation to the new host can stimulate modifications of virus phenotype and expansion into new ecological niches, eventually giving rise to "new" hantaviruses sufficiently distinct that are able to exploit new geographical areas. At least three instances of this happening have now been recorded. Nemirov et al. (2002) have examined the phylogenetic trees of hantaviruses and compared these to the D-loop region of mitochondrial DNA. These studies show a remarkable concordance between murine evolution and the evolution of hantaviruses. Focusing on the divergence of Saaremaa virus from Dobrava virus, Nemirov et al. have speculated that Saaremaa virus has evolved as a result of Dobrava virus switching host from the yellow-striped field mouse (*Apodemus flavicollis*) to *A. agrarius*, the striped field mouse. The result is a virus with a reduced pathogenicity for humans compared to Dubrova virus, although there are some qualifications as to just how pathogenic the latter virus really is. Other examples include transmission of Monongahella virus from *Peromyscus maniculatus* to *P. leucopus*, eventually leading to the evolution of New York virus (Morzunov et al., 1998). A second example is Puumala virus from *Clethrionomys* "host-switching" species to *Lemmus* and then onto *Microtus* species, thence establishing lineages to the present day Topografov and Khabarovsk viruses (Vapalahti et al., 1999b).

In general, phylogenetic trees constructed using L, M or S RNA genomic sequences are the same, suggesting a similar evolution for all three RNA segments (Nemirov et al., 1999). Hantavirus evolution resembles that of an extrachromosal genetic element of murines rather more than it does of that of an autonomous, horizontally transmitted agent (Hjelle and Yates, 2001).

Epidemiology

Hantavirus disease in humans first became recognised during the Korean conflict in 1951–1952. A new disease, called Korean haemorrhagic fever, was seen in over 2000 soldiers serving with the United Nation forces (Earle, 1954). Since its discovery, the disease caused by Hantaan virus has been referred to by a wide variety of names, for example epidemic haemorrhagic fever. Other names were coined throughout Asia and Europe, influenced by various regional preferences for naming the disease. Collectively, all of these various syndromes are now referred to as HFRS.

A less severe form of HFRS—originally termed nephropathia endemica—is found in Scandinavia, the Baltic States, Eastern Europe, the Balkans, and Greece, as well as throughout the former Soviet Union. Detailed descriptions of neuropathia endemica have been available since the 1930s. The similarities between this disease and that found in Asia became apparent as work with Hantaan virus advanced sufficiently to the point that diagnostic reagents became readily available, this in turn opening up the possibility of detailed epidemiological and pathological studies.

Human hantavirus disease in Asia is very much linked to the ecology and biology of its rodent host, *A. agrarius*. As a result, there is marked seasonality in the number of human infections, most cases occurring in the autumn and early winter months when rodent numbers are at their peak and harvesting is underway. Hantaan virus is responsible annually for over 100,000 cases in the People's Republic of China, a number that almost certainly is a gross underestimate of its true incidence.

Those most at risk of infection are those individuals who may come into contact with rodents and rodent excreta on a regular basis. This can be by virtue of their occupation, living conditions or lifestyle. Abundant evidence from Korea and elsewhere in Asia has confirmed that agricultural workers are at greatest risk, particularly when food production is labour intensive. In parts of Europe, forestry employees, hunters and those engaged in trapping wild mammals all show a higher incidence of infection compared to other individuals (Groen et al., 1995; Vapalahti et al., 1999a).

The emergence of HPS in the 1990s led to a renewed effort in identifying risk factors. The cleaning of food stores and agricultural outbuildings was identified as an additional high risk activity particularly if the buildings had been closed and left unventilated for any length of time (Zeitz et al., 1995, 1997; Van Loock et al., 1999).

Diagnosis

Laboratory diagnosis is critically dependent upon serology as the viraemia is short lived and thus the chance of detecting virus is low. Reverse transcriptase PCR can be employed to detect viral genomes, and indeed the use of PCR is essential if genotype comparisons and a definitive diagnosis are to be arrived at as to the involvement of a particular hantavirus. However, positive reactions using acute phase sera by RT-PCR are achieved in a maximum of 70% of cases, although often success is less than 50%. As is always the case in viral diagnosis, RT-PCR is not recommended as a sole diagnostic test because of the considerable risk of cross-contamination. Generally with RNA viruses the necessity of performing a reverse transcription step prior to the PCR reaction also presents difficulties in estimating the number of viral genomes, and thus linking virus burden to disease severity cannot be undertaken easily.

Ideally, virus isolation is desirable for a definitive diagnosis, but with hantaviruses there is a major problem as these viruses, for reasons yet to be determined, do not grow readily in cell culture. Vero E6 cells (a clone of a commonly used line of African Monkey Kidney cells) are used routinely for isolation and growth of virus stocks, but fresh isolates often require repeated serial passage before plaques can be seen under an agar overlay. Thus, there is a risk that such virus stocks no longer accurately represent the sequence of epitopes critical for detecting neutralising antibodies, although it has to be said that Chizhikov et al. (1995) did not find any evidence of amino acid substitutions in an isolate of Sin Nombre Virus originally derived from lung tissue and previously passaged in E6 cells.

By far the most useful diagnostic tests are those designed for detecting hantavirus-specific IgM antibodies using either immunofluorescence or a more sensitive ELISA (Padula et al., 2000a). IgM antibodies are present early in the acute phase and can be detected throughout all phases and well into convalescence. Most of the early IgM antibody response during acute infection is directed against epitopes on the nucleocapsid (N) protein, with this response declining rapidly in the weeks following recovery. Recombinant proteins can be used, most readily by expression of the N protein in insect cells.[2] Detection of IgM is particularly appropriate against a background of low exposure amongst the local population, but can be more problematical in regions such as South America, where exposure is clearly that much greater. In Paraguay, for example, a seroprevalence level approaching 40% has been found in the general population (Peters, 1998). The possibility of non-specific cross-reactions can be minimised using a format that does not rely on direct IgM binding to the solid phase coated with viral antigen.

Neutralising IgG antibodies are detected as early as the first week of acute infection and may last for many years. From the diagnostic point of view, it is increasingly clear that the use of a single antigen may be insufficient to provide an accurate and reliable diagnosis should several hantaviruses be circulating in the same environment, especially in Europe and Asia. For example, although Hantaan and Dobrava nucleocapsid proteins show a high degree of cross-reactivity for human antibodies, Dobrava antigen only detects 76% of Hantaan-specific sera (Brus et al., 2000). Therefore, tests for IgG antibodies need to incorporate at least three antigens, those of Hantaan, Dobrava and Puumala viruses, if not also that of Seoul virus as a fourth (Hujakka et al., 2003). Serodiagnosis using immunoblot assays incorporating a number of different antigens representative of New World hantavirus has been used to good effect (Hjelle et al., 1997).

It is likely that IgG antibodies protect against secondary infection (Padula et al., 2000b; Settergren et al., 1991), but it is not known as to the extent of cross-protection against heterologous hantaviruses. Given the high level of exposure to hantaviruses in places such as the Balkans and South America, this could be an important issue. Neither is it known to what extent secondary exposure may be relied upon to boost antibody levels.

Differential diagnosis is difficult for both HFRS and HPS. The early signs of HFRS can easily be confused with leptospirosis, typhus, streptococcal glomerulonephritis or pyelonephritis. Mild cases of HFRS can be confused with streptococcal pharyngitis, influenza, hepatitis A or non-steroidal anti-inflammatory activity. HPS is extremely difficult to tell apart from influenza in its early stages. Thrombocytopenia is an important clinical feature of human infections, and therefore evidence of reduced platelet activity is a must in order to eliminate other possible causes of acute respiratory distress. However, a fever coupled with a thrombocytopenia, together with an increased number of circulating immature neutrophils and lymphoblasts, is pathognomic of HPS.

Clinical profiles

The typical acute infection in Asian patients generally progresses through a number of clinically well-defined phases. Most of the clinical symptoms result from the underlying

---

[2] Reagents are available from the Centres for Disease Control, Atlanta, USA for the formatting of these tests, and there are several commercial manufacturers (e.g. Progen Diagnostics, Heidelberg, Germany; Focus Technologies, Cypress, California, USA; Mikrogen, Martinsreid, Germany).

Table 3

Disease progression in humans with haemorrhagic fever with renal syndrome (HFRS)

Phase	Description	Duration	Features
1	Febrile	3–7 days	Fever, chills; malaise; nausea; abdominal pain. Virus isolation difficult
2	Hypotensive	2–48 h	Thrombocytopenia; first evidence of haemorrhage in severe cases
3	Oliguric	3–7 days	Renal failure; proteinuria; high levels of serum creatinine and urea. Blood pressure returns to normal in later days in survivors
4	Diuretic	Days to weeks	Heavy diuresis; length possibly related to disease severity
5	Convalescent	Weeks	Normally complete, with few if any adverse effects

renal pathology, this ranging from renal dysfunction to renal failure. The five recognised phases are in order of occurrence: febrile, hypotensive, oliguria, diuretic and convalescence (Table 3) (Davies et al., 1985).

Haemorrhagic fever with renal syndrome

The term "haemorrhagic fever with renal disease syndrome" was first proposed by Nobel laureate Carlton Gajdusek (Gajdusek, 1962) in an attempt to consolidate the numerous clinical descriptions of disease into a common descriptor. The World Health Organisation eventually endorsed this nomenclature in 1983 to embrace the global spectrum of clinical manifestations that we now associate with hantaviruses. It needs to be borne in mind, however, that the vast majority of infections caused by these viruses do not give overt signs of bleeding or internal haemorrhage.

The clinical course of the disease is usually described as consisting of up to five phases (Table 3). As with most infections described in this book, the onset tends to be sudden after an incubation period of up to 4 weeks. Patients present with a spectrum of symptoms including fever, malaise, nausea and general abdominal pain. This febrile first stage lasts up to 7 days when signs of petechiae and conjunctival haemorrhages presage the second, hypotensive phase. This stage lasts from as short as a few hours or up to 2 days with a marked thrombocytopenia being the major clinical indication of underlying disease development. In severe cases—most notably in Hantaan and Dobrava virus infections—the patients enter quickly into a state of hypovolemic shock, such instances accounting for nearly a third of total deaths from hantavirus infections. Thus, there is considerable prognostic importance in determining the nature of the causative virus within a week of onset, although this may be difficult as the brief viraemia in the early days of the first stage mitigates against a successful sequencing of the viral RNA.

Those patients surviving the second stage go on to quickly display signs of renal impairment. This third, oliguric stage is characterised by all the signs of severe renal disease, which may prove fatal in up to 50% of cases. A massive proteinuria is paralleled by elevated levels of serum creatinine and urea. For those cases that overcome the oliguric stage, there follows a return to normal blood pressure within 7 days and is followed by a fourth, diuretic phase, the length of which some investigators have suggested is determined by the severity of the preceding phases.

Convalescence usually is complete, although this may take several weeks. The phases are most significant in cases from Asia, the far eastern regions of the former Soviet Union and the Balkans, but can be hard to discern as the disease takes its course. Clinicians have particularly difficulty in differentiating urban cases from other causes of influenza-like illness, especially if the infection is due to Seoul virus, normally linked with a more mild clinical illness. As a consequence numerous cases, especially in Asia, are most likely to go unrecognised.

European investigators have been concerned with cases of what was previously referred to as nephropathia endemica for over 70 years, and thus there are many detailed clinical descriptions in the literature of cases due to hantaviruses more prevalent in Scandinavia and Eastern Europe. In particular, nephropathia endemica is associated with Puumala virus infection which has a case fatality rate of below 1% and rarely presents with signs of haemorrhage (Lee and van der, 1989).

Hantavirus pulmonary syndrome

The disease is characterised by a prodromal phase of 3–5 days in which the patient complains of myalgia, malaise and a fever that starts abruptly. Noticeably a cough and coriza is absent. Onset of acute illness begins 14–17 days after exposure, heralded by abdominal pain, nausea and vomiting. Records kept at CDC indicate that patients at this stage are likely to seek medical aid but up to half are given palliative therapy and sent home (Peters and Khan, 2002). However, if there are grounds to suspect hantavirus infection, especially if patient lifestyle and area of residence indicate a close proximity to rodents, a simple blood smear is sufficient to indicate whether or not a thrombocytopenia is present.

By the time patients are hospitalised they have often developed cardiopulmonary and gastrointestinal involvement. Tachycardia, tachypnea and postural hypotension are present although a chest examination does not give much of an indication, with only a few rales detected. A declining platelet count and the appearance of atypical lymphocytes distinguish the acute phase from other infectious diseases with similar prodromal symptoms, particularly plague, tularaemia, relapsing fever and chlamydial infections. Pulmonary involvement is manifested by a low pO_2 level or low pulse oximetry findings, often with hypocapnia. Chest radiographs show all patients to have extensive interstitial oedema within 48 h after admission, with at least two-thirds showing signs of extensive airway disease accompanied by pleural effusion. Importantly, these findings contrast with those seen in patients with other acute respiratory diseases.

Clinical experience since the initial Four Corners outbreak shows that patient management in severe cases is made the more difficult by the increase in pulmonary vascular permeability in the face of myocardial dysfunction. Thus, treatment is a matter of balancing cardiac output with the need to reduce pulmonary oedema. The use of inotropic drugs such as dobutamine has been recommended and should be given as early as possible (Hallin et al., 1996). However, 30–40% of patients die within 24–48 h after admission, even if admitted to the best of intensive care units. These severe cases show evidence of disseminated intravascular coagulation and haemorrhage plus elevated levels of lymphocytes. The degree of thrombocytopenia is a critical prognostic marker, mortality being directly correlated with loss of platelets (Zaki et al., 1995; Nolte et al., 1995).

Importantly, there is no absolute demarcation between the clinical course in patients with hantavirus pulmonary syndrome and corresponding cases of haemorrhagic fever with renal syndrome. As has been shown for Andes virus, cases of HPS can include a renal pathology and there are reports of HFRS patients with additional involvement of the lungs.

Pathology

Generally it is thought that hantaviruses are not cytolytic for endothelial cells with monocytes representing the primary sites of infection. The pathology of hantavirus infections is likely to be largely the result of an activated immune response. This is supported by the finding of activated CD8 + T cells circulating in patients with HFRS (Huang et al., 1994) and a CTL infiltrate in kidney tissues from individuals with Puumala virus infection (Temonen et al., 1996). Activated CD8 + cells have also been found in patients with HPS (Nolte et al., 1995). Memory T cells can be found in individuals infected with Puumala virus up to 15 years previously (Van Epps et al., 1999). Memory T cells directed against a single epitope on N protein reached levels of 100–300 per 10^6 PBMCs, comparable to the levels seen in patients with acute influenza or measles virus infection, despite the elapse of at least 6 years since the loss of Puumala virus. Overall, the specificity of the immune response has been found as polyclonal, directed against at least six epitopes on N, the profile dependent upon the HLA haplotype of the donor (Van Epps et al., 1999) Fig. 6. Only 3 out of 22 cytotoxic T cell lines generated in this study were cross-reactive for Hantaan or Sin Nombre Virus, suggesting the long-lived memory responses are highly specific for Puumala virus.

There was no evidence of continuing Puumala virus infection in any of the 13 Finnish patients that were central to this study, suggesting immunological memory was retained over long periods of time without the need for periodic re-stimulation. This is in accord with the work of Ahmed and colleagues (Lau et al., 1994; Murali-Krishna et al., 1999) who demonstrated that CD8 + T cells directed against LCM virus could be successfully transferred into naïve wild-type or class I-deficient mice.

Hantaviruses enter endothelial cells and monocytes by binding to β3 integrin (CD61) (Gavrilovskaya et al., 1999). The strong activated T cell response depends critically on the capture of hantaviruses by immature dendritic cells in the epithelium and interstitium of the lungs. These process viral proteins to present peptides associated with MHC

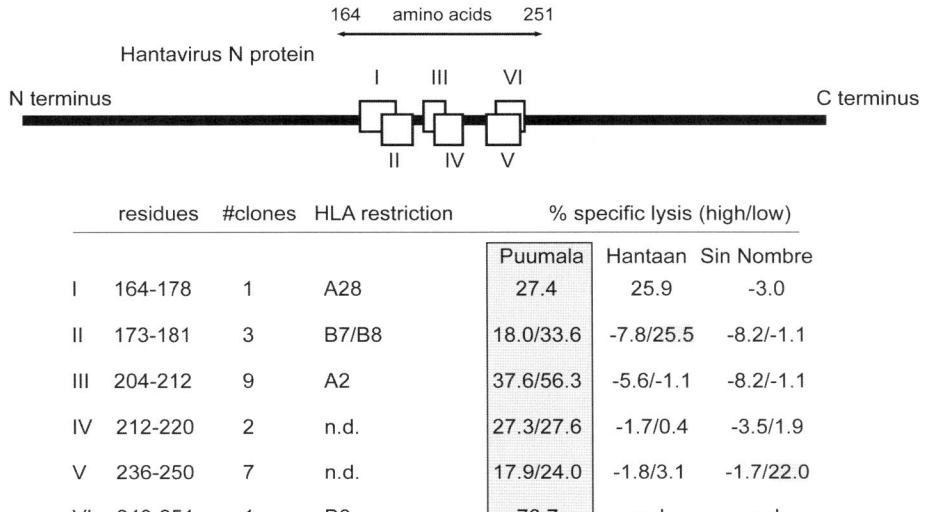

Fig. 6 Mapping of class I immune responses in humans infected with hantaviruses (data from Van Epps et al., 2002).

molecules on the cell surface. Raftery et al. (2002) have shown that hantaviruses can successfully replicate in dendritic cells in a non-cytolytic manner. Importantly, infected dendritic cells activate resting T cells just as effectively as uninfected dendritic cells. Infection leads to release of TNFα which could mirror the high levels of this cytokine found both in HFRS patients (Linderholm et al., 1996; Temonen et al., 1996) and in those infected with Puumala virus (Kanerva et al., 1998). In this context, it has been reported that 42% of patients hospitalised with HFRS have the less common TNF2 allele in the promoter region of the TNFα gene as opposed to 15% of healthy controls (Kanerva et al., 1998).

There is some evidence suggesting disease severity is related to the HLA type of the patient. Mustonen and colleagues have reported that among 74 Finnish cases of HFRS due to Puumala virus there was a significant linkage between HLA haplotype B8 DRB1*0301 and severe renal impairment or signs of shock. Such patients have also been described as supporting higher levels of virus replication (Plyusnin et al., 1997). In contrast, the same workers have shown less than half of the expected numbers of patients with mild disease possessed the HLA B27 allele (Mustonen et al., 1998). This linkage is noted by the authors as being akin to that seen between HLA haplotype and disease progression in patients with HIV.

Treatment

Until recently neither prophylactic nor chemotherapeutic agents were available for the prevention and treatment of hantavirus infections, despite being one of the most important causes of morbidity and mortality in the Republic of Korea and parts of the People's Republic of China.

Antiviral therapy

As with the treatment of many haemorrhagic fevers, ribavirin has received serious attention (Andrei and De Clercq, 1993). *In vitro* studies have shown that ribavirin inhibits Seoul virus replication (Murphy et al., 2000), with the error rate of hantavirus RNA synthesis increased nearly ninefold, equivalent to four base substitutions per S RNA segment (Severson et al., 2003). Up to eight random insertions occurred, suggesting polymerase slippage. Thus, during replication new viral RNA molecules become increasingly devoid of genetic information and mRNA molecules thus generated fail to be translated into viral protein. Ribavirin has been shown to have some benefit in the treatment of HFRS. In a fully controlled, double blind study centred on 242 patients in China, administration of ribavirin significantly lessened the risk of patients progressing to the oliguric phase and shock, and reduced overall the number of case fatalities (Huggins et al., 1991).

In contrast, intravenous administration of ribavirin to patients with HPS has proved disappointing (Chapman et al., 1999). High doses of corticosteroids have also been considered in South American patients but as with all anecdotal intervention strategies there is a lack of controlled trials and a paucity of follow-up data.

Interferon is known to inhibit virus replication *in vitro* and *in vivo*. Tamura and colleagues demonstrated a reduction in the titre of Hantaan virus grown in E6 cells and treatment of infected suckling mice with interferon-β prolonged the survival time. Further indications as to its potential for treating HFRS were had by noticing the prolonged survival time in suckling mice infected with Hantaan virus (Tamura et al., 1987). More recent studies have shown that interferon will inhibit Puumala virus growth in macrophages in a dose-dependent manner (Temonen et al., 1995). The role of macrophages is likely complex, however, as the same study showed that mature macrophages became less resistant to Puumala virus and thus may aid virus dissemination *in vivo*. If Puumala virus is representative of other hantaviruses, then these viruses are poor inducers of interferon, and any observed inhibition is not linked with MxA protein activity, a GTPase and one of the principal antiviral inhibitors induced by the interferons.

Vaccine development

In 1984 the World Health Organisation recommended the development of an effective inactivated vaccine as a matter of priority. One such product (Hantavax) has been prepared and undergone limited efficacy studies in Korea (Cho and Howard, 1999). This

Hantaan virus vaccine is prepared from the ROK 84-105 Hantaan virus strain by growth in suckling mouse brain. This strain was originally isolated from a patient in the early acute stage of HFRS using Vero E-6 cells. Immunisation with this formalin-inactivated vaccine resulted in 97% seroconversion for IgG, and 75% seroconversion for neutralising antibodies, after two intramuscular doses. A booster dose at 12 months showed a good anamnestic response for total IgG levels but the development of neutralising antibodies was less impressive, with only 50% of volunteers positive by the plaque reduction test 1 month after the booster dose. This suggests that the classical approach of two or three doses initially followed by a boost up to a year later is not ideal: the inactivation process may destroy critical B-cell determinants or the adjuvant may not be stimulating expansion of the critical B-cell populations required for sustained protective immunity.

Similar efforts in Japan have also focused on the development of an inactivated vaccine, using the Seoul B-1 strain previously passaged 26 times in new-born ICR mice brains (Yamanishi et al., 1988). There is some concern as to the choice of the B-1 strain, however, as this virus was originally isolated from an infected rat using a malignant tumour cell line, not the ideal pedigree for a product designed for human use.

Given the immensity of the public health problem of HFRS in China, there have been a number of attempts to produce a vaccine suitable for its control. Song et al. (1992) developed an attenuated, monovalent golden hamster kidney cell culture vaccine that was attenuated sufficiently for human use. Little has been reported as to its evaluation in clinical trials, however. In a separate Chinese study, nearly 2500 volunteers were reported to have been injected with a formalin-inactivated vaccine (Zhu et al., 1994). Seroconversion rates were similar to those reported by Cho and Howard (1999) for Hantavax. Again, a boost at 12 months only marginally elevated neutralising antibody titres. That a significant secondary response can be obtained was shown by Lu et al. (1996) who found those exposed to the virus developed an anamnestic response after having received just one dose of inactivated vaccine.

A vaccinia-vectored vaccine has been produced by the US Department of Defense. This vector expresses both envelope glycoproteins (Gn and Gc) as well as the internal nucleocapsid protein (N) (Schmaljohn et al., 1990). This recombinant vector performed well in a hamster challenge study, and the immunogen was superior to hantavirus proteins expressed in the baculovirus system. Importantly, protection was passively transferred by antibody to these immunogens, suggesting that a B cell response may be sufficient for protection in humans. This vaccine has been extensively purified with a view to its eventual peripheral use, thus avoiding the problems of generalised vaccine reactions and spread to non-immunised contacts, always a concern when using vaccinia as a vector (McClain et al., 2000). In phase I trials, subcutaneous injection of 10^7 plaque forming units proved superior to scarification for inducing vaccinia virus immunity. The subsequent phase II study comprising 142 volunteers was carried out using two injections 4 weeks apart. Neutralising antibodies were found in 98% after the second dose, but in substantially fewer (28%) of volunteers with previously acquired immunity to vaccinia.

Although hantaviruses can infect several species of non-human primates, the infection is asymptomatic, with a mild proteinuria and elevated transaminases being the only signs of disease. Newborn mice can support hantavirus replication, but susceptibility declines rapidly with age, thus preventing any meaningful studies in adult animals, such as the testing of candidate vaccine immunogens. This, of course, raises the side issue as to how feral rodent populations become persistently infected.

As an alternative, Hooper et al. (2001) have investigated the use of Syrian hamsters. This species proved unexpectedly useful; studies revealed that Andes virus was lethal for adult hamsters but Sin Nombre virus was not. Up to 93% of animals succumbed to Andes virus infection with all the signs of a subacute interstitial pneumonia and accompanying pleural effusion, both features of human HPS. In contrast to human infections, however, there were signs of a subacute hepatitis. Furthermore, virus could be cultivated from infected tissues, something that has proven difficult using material from human cases obtained at autopsy. The value of this research was enhanced by asking the question as to what extent prior exposure of hamsters to heterologous, non-pathogenic hantaviruses could protect against a subsequent lethal challenge of Andes virus. The answer was that animals were protected but this protection was not directly the result of the production of neutralising antibodies directed against the immunising, heterologous virus. The implication is that class I MHC mediated responses are likely to play an important role in protective immunity, at least in this animal model. If confirmed, this would require a re-evaluation of the precept that antibody alone is sufficient to confer protection against a bunyavirus infection.

Hantaviruses and history

The emergence of hantaviruses, in particular the pulmonary syndrome (HPS) associated with the Sin Nombre Virus, has led to a reawakening among medical historians as to the probable cause of illnesses that emerged in centuries past, only to mysteriously disappear before modern times. In particular, there is a remarkable similarity in primary sources between modern descriptions of human hantavirus disease and the sweating sickness (*Sudor Anglicus*) of Tudor England. "The sweats" likely caused at least five epidemics during the reigns of Henry VII and Henry VIII. First recorded shortly after Henry VII gained the English crown on Bosworth Field in 1485, John Caius described the illness in some detail as having a sudden onset, characterised by fever, headache, limb pain, malaise and profuse sweating, as well as tachycardia and other cardiac signs (Holmes, 1998). Apart from the sweating, this is somewhat similar in outline to the clinical description of the patients seen during the Four Corners outbreak in 1993. Both afflict more males than females, although this may simply reflect an increased risk of exposure to the host reservoir. A crucial difference is the question of human-to-human transmission. This is not a contributory feature of hantavirus epidemics, although there is evidence of human transmission of hantavirus (Andes virus) in Argentina and Chile.

There has been considerable speculation as to the probable causative agent of "the sweats". At various times sweating sickness has been ascribed to infectious agents as diverse as enterovirus, arbovirus and relapsing fever. Wylie and Collier (1981) favoured influenza, although the seasonality of the outbreaks and what we know of its epidemiology makes the linkage with influenza less likely.

Wylie and Collier proposed that sweating sickness originated in Siberia, spread across Russia and into the Baltic States, from where it was carried to northern England in cargoes of fur and timber. This plausible scenario would infer the introduction of infected rodents into the British Isles followed by spread of the disease southward as supporters of the Tudor monarchy established themselves in and around London. Alternatively, it could have been introduced into England when Henry Tudor landed in Wales in 1483 with a small French army and spread when he subsequently dispatched Richard III at Bosworth Field. Whether it came from France or from the ports of northeast England, it arrived in London in August that same year. We know that the summer of 1485 was particularly wet and warm, ideal conditions for the rapid expansion of rodent numbers. It is worth recalling that such climatic factors also played a role in elevating dramatically the rodent of host of the Sin Nombre virus during the Four Corners outbreak in 1993. Thus in Tudor England urban outbreaks occurred when rodents increased to a level sufficient to penetrate cities and towns. The supposition is that town dwellers, unlike their country cousins, had not been exposed to the agent sufficiently early in life to have developed immunity as a result of asymptomatic infections in childhood. Holmes has,

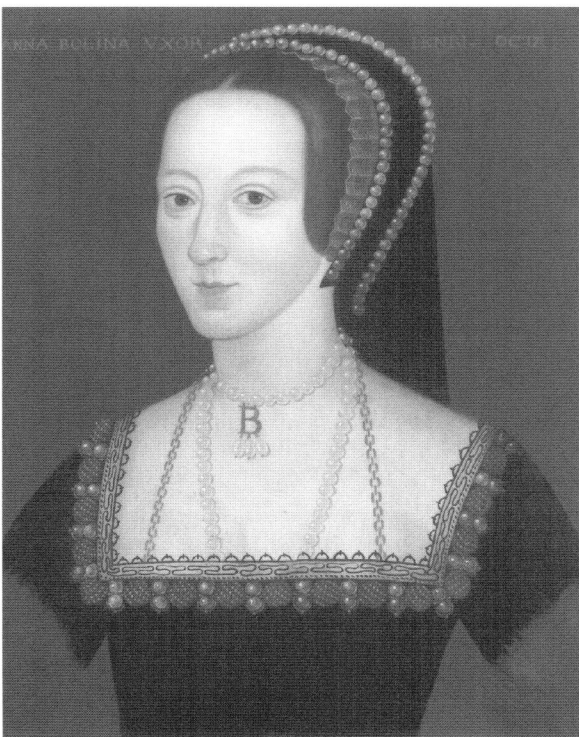

Fig. 7 Anne Boleyn (1501–1536), second wife of Henry VIII of England, recorded as suffering "the sweats" in 1528 (photograph courtesy of the National Portrait Gallery, London).

quite plausibly, suggested that the virus remained endemic in the countryside at this time. There is some evidence contemporary evidence to support this theory: anti-hantavirus antibody prevalence in country areas is higher in the US east coast among both adults and children.

After its first appearance in 1485, the sweating sickness caused severe epidemics in 1508, 1517, 1528 and finally in 1551. Dyer (1997) has scrutinised English parish records and concluded that "the sweats" accounted for around 15,000 deaths at a time when the population of England was about three million. As in contemporary times, it was the suddenness of disease onset by hitherto something unknown that instilled fear and panic, particularly among town dwellers. These figures are comparatively low, however, when compared to the 30,000 deaths from plague in 1563 and 180,000 deaths from influenza from 1557 to 1559 (Bridson, 2001). The epidemic of 1528 was particularly virulent, affecting the corridors of power (Fig. 7). The Archbishop of Canterbury lost 14 of his staff to the sweating sickness and it caused Henry VIII to temporarily abandon his future second wife, Anne Boleyn, when she and her father succumbed (Holmes, 1998).

Whether or not sweating sickness was due to some mediaeval ancestor of present-day hantaviruses, it serves to illustrate that the concept of emerging infections is not new. Mass movement of people and the disruption of war introduce new threats that often account for a greater loss of life than military action. Little has changed in this respect over the last 500 years.

Summary

Crimean-Congo haemorrhagic fever causes the most extensive haemorrhagic manifestations. Its occurrence is widespread from Central Africa through central and eastern Europe to north-west China. It has the interesting molecular property of coding for an L RNA segment product approximately twice the length of similar polymerases encoded by the genomes of Rift Valley fever or hantaviruses. Sporadic outbreaks of Rift Valley fever continue to occur, increasingly in areas that were previously free of disease. Many consider Rift Valley fever as a particular threat to Europe and the Americas, not least because it is a significant pathogen of man and animals. Integration between medical and

Table 4

Bunyaviruses—key questions

What is the significance of the large L protein encoded by the Crimean-Congo haemorrhagic fever virus, and is this related to its pathology?

How can experience with Rift Valley virus vaccines for veterinary use be translated into developing products for use in humans?

Is antibody alone sufficient to confer protection?

What is the underlying molecular basis for the spectrum of disease caused by hantaviruses?

Is the emergence of Garissa virus an isolated instance or does it represent a readiness for reassortment between bunyaviruses co-circulating in animal and livestock populations?

---

veterinary surveillance agencies is thus critical, as animal deaths may go unrecorded until human cases are reported. The emergence of Garissa virus is a cause for concern, representing as it does a potentially new threat to large parts of East Africa and elsewhere, doubly so as it may occur simultaneously with Rift Valley fever. Climatic changes significantly affect the incidence of bunyavirus-induced haemorrhagic disease. Abnormal rainfall patterns led to the emergence of Sin Nombre virus in 1993 and over the ensuing decade it has become clear that there is a completely new genre of hantavirus with the propensity to cause severe respiratory illness throughout the Americas. With all of these viruses, control measures require a balance between co-ordinated surveillance, vector and rodent control and clinicians alert for the first signs of anything unusual in terms of case presentation. Prospects for vaccination and therapy, although not adequate, are considerably better than is the case for other causes of viral haemorrhagic disease.

Filoviruses

The filovirus family has at present only two discrete members, Marburg and Ebola viruses. There are at least four serotypes of Ebola viruses, with the Reston virus frequently referred to as a separate viral species. Both Marburg and Ebola are indigenous to Africa and cause severe haemorrhagic disease in man and non-human primates. The discovery of the Reston agent in monkeys imported into the United States led to the realisation that Ebola-like agents may be lurking in other parts of the world including Asia as well as in Africa. Non-human primates are highly susceptible to the African serotypes of Ebola virus, in particular the large apes. There is every indication that gorilla families have been particularly hard hit by devastating outbreaks of Ebola over the past decade.

Initial studies on these agents suggested morphology similar to that of the rhabdoviruses, but both agents were later shown to possess features distinctive enough to warrant the proposal of a new virus family, the Filoviridae. The name refers to the long filamentous appearance of these viruses under the electron microscope (Latin: filo = filament or thread). Filoviruses share a similar genetic organisation with the members of the families Paramyxoviridae and Rhabdoviridae. The three families have recently been grouped into a single taxonomic order, the Mononegavirales.[1]

The names of filoviruses refer to the places where they were first recorded; in 1967 outbreaks of haemorrhagic fever occurred in three places in Europe, including Marburg, Germany, among handlers of tissue from imported African green monkeys. In 1976, two epidemics occurred simultaneously in southern Sudan and across the border in the north of what is now the Democratic Republic of the Congo.[2] Although these latter outbreaks are now known to have been due to viruses with somewhat different properties, both were referred to as Ebola after a small river to the north of Yambuku, the home of the patient in Zaire from whom the first isolate was obtained. There has since been evidence of filovirus infections in neighbouring regions and in other parts of Africa as far apart as Liberia and Zimbabwe (Table 1). A series of outbreaks varying in intensity continues to occur in central Africa, the most notable being the 1995 outbreak centred on the Congolese city of Kikwit. A new form of Ebola, named Reston after the locality in Virginia, USA where it first came to light, has been associated with cynomolgus monkeys (*Macaca fascicularis*) first imported in the Philippines. It is reasonable to assume that other filoviruses may exist in Africa and elsewhere which may initially be mistaken for alternative causes of haemorrhagic fever. The Reston outbreak did much to influence public interest

---

[1] See http://www.ncbi.nlm.nih.gov/ICTVdb for a full description.
[2] For the sake of clarity, the older name of Zaire is retained in this book where the name refers to particular isolates of virus or virus strains.

Table 1

Recorded outbreaks of filovirus infections, 1997–2003

Virus	Year	Location	Cases	Mortality
Marburg	1967	West Germany	29	7 (23%)
	1967	Yugoslavia	2	0
	1975	Southern Africa	3	1 (33%)
	1980	Kenya	2	1 (50%)
	1982	South Africa	1	0
	1987	Kenya	1	1
Ebola	1972	Zaire	1[a]	0
	1976	Sudan	360	150 (42%)
	1976	Zaire	237	211 (89%)
	1977	Zaire	2	2
	1979	Sudan	34	22 (65%)
	1994	Gabon	44	29 (63%)
	1995	Côte d'Ivoire	1	0
	1995	Zaire	315	244 (77%)
	1995	Côte d'Ivoire	1	0
	1996	Gabon	37	21 (57%)
	1996	Gabon	60	45 (75%)
	2000	Uganda	315	217 (69%)
	2002	Gabon	60	50 (83%)
	2002	Congo[b]	143	128 (90%)
	2003	Congo	31	29[c] (94%)
Ebola (Reston)	1989	USA	4[d]	0
	1990	Philippines	12[d]	0
	1992	Italy	0[d]	0

[a]Retrospective diagnosis.
[b]Democratic Republic of Congo: formerly Zaire.
[c]As of 11 December 2003.
[d]Monkeys.

in dangerous pathogens, culminating in the movie "Outbreak" based on the popular book "The Hot Zone" by Preston (1994). This described in graphic detail how the Reston outbreak was first identified and the measures taken. Importantly, it recalls the pressures scientists can be placed under by the media at a time when their preoccupations are containment and control.

There are a number of specialist collections of articles that give a good overview of what is known as the epidemiology and pathology of human filovirus infections. Although published over 40 years ago, the monograph edited by Martini and Siegert (1971) contains useful early descriptions of the cases of Marburg virus infections. A further symposium volume edited by Pattyn (1978) likewise contains early information as to the Ebola virus outbreaks of 1997. For more recent overviews, the 1999 special issue of Journal of Infectious Diseases (vol. 179, Suppl. 1) should be consulted. These are complemented by recent reviews of the strides that have been made in understanding the molecular properties of these viruses, for example Feldmann et al. (2001), and approaches toward vaccine development (Feldmann et al., 2003).

Epidemiology

Despite the infamous reputation of Ebola and Marburg viruses, all outbreaks until recently have been self-limiting, with the total number of recorded fatalities over the last three decades still below a few thousand. The situation is most likely changing, however, as there have been prolonged outbreaks of Ebola in Gabon and other parts of central Africa since 1995. Outbreaks of human filovirus infection invariably occur in or at the end of the tropical rainy season. All index cases have been in persons living close to tropical rain forests or in the marginal zone between forest and savannah. Although widely regarded as a zoonosis, the animal reservoir(s) of the filoviruses have eluded discovery (see below).

A feature common to both Marburg and Ebola is transmission by close contact. Disease is spread rapidly via contaminated needles and other sharp instruments. Almost certainly virus can be sexually transmitted. Of all viruses to infect humans, only rabies is known to have a greater mortality for humans.

Marburg virus

Marburg disease, erroneously referred to in the popular press as African green monkey disease, was first recognised in 1967, when it caused three simultaneous outbreaks in Europe among workers producing kidney cell cultures for the production of poliovirus vaccines: at Marburg, Frankfurt and Belgrade (Martini, 1973). There were 31 cases, of which 25 were primary infections; seven of the primary cases died, but there were no deaths among the six secondary cases. A hitherto unknown virus was isolated. All the primary cases were laboratory staff who had come into direct contact with blood, organs or tissue cultures from one particular consignment of vervet monkeys (*Cercopithecus aethiops*) imported from Uganda. Four secondary infections were hospital personnel who had come into close contact with patients' blood. The wife of a Yugoslav veterinary surgeon was infected through blood contact with her husband, and a further patient transmitted the disease to his wife during sexual intercourse 83 days after the onset of illness. Marburg virus was detected in his seminal fluid. Fortunately there were no tertiary cases and the virus did not spread into the community.

The disease next appeared in 1975. A young Australian man who had been hitchhiking through central and southern Africa died shortly after admission to a Johannesburg hospital. His female travelling companion and a nurse who looked after him also contracted the disease. Both women survived. Virological investigations confirmed that the virus isolated from all three cases was morphologically and antigenically identical to the Marburg virus isolated in Germany some years earlier.

In 1980, Marburg virus reappeared, this time in Kenya. A 58-year-old engineer was admitted to a Nairobi hospital with an 8-day history of progressive fever, myalgia and backache. By the time the patient was admitted, he was in peripheral vascular failure and bleeding profusely from the gastrointestinal tract. He died within 6 h of admission. Marburg virus particles were seen by electron microscopy in liver and kidney tissues removed at post-mortem. Nine days later a doctor who had attended this patient and who had attempted resuscitation became ill with a similar syndrome. He survived, and Marburg infection was confirmed serologically.

A fourth occurrence was an isolated case recognised during a routine surveillance programme in Kenya undertaken in 1987 (Johnson et al., 1996). This case is of particular interest as it was found close to the area from where the vervet monkeys were trapped that subsequently caused the 1967 outbreak in Europe.

Ebola virus

Between June and November 1976, outbreaks of a severe and often fatal haemorrhagic fever occurred in the equatorial provinces of the Sudan and Zaire (Fig. 1). In Sudan there were 284 known cases, with a case fatality rate of 53%. The numbers succumbing were greater at 88% among the 318 cases in Zaire. The viruses isolated from patients in both these outbreaks were found to be morphologically identical with Marburg virus yet antigenically distinct.

The outbreaks in Zaire centred around a Catholic mission run by the Sisters of the Holy Heart of Maria in the remote northern village of Yambuku. The first recorded case,

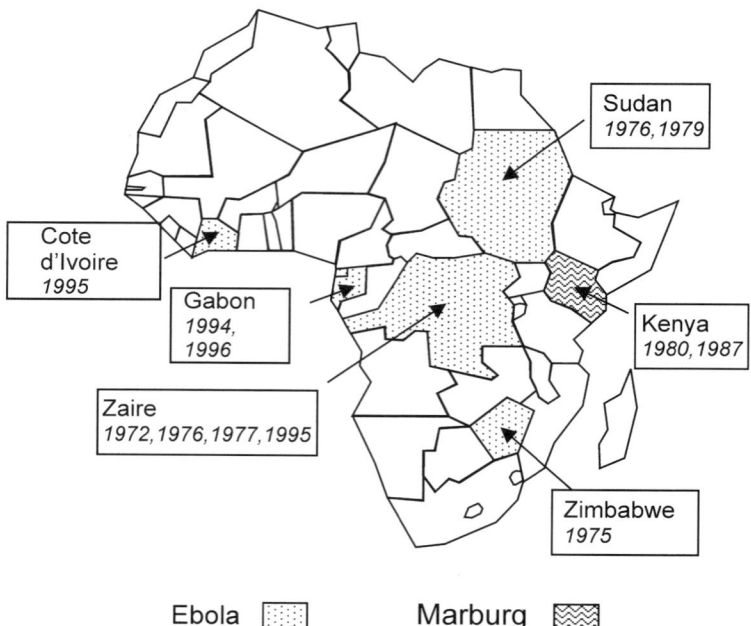

Fig. 1 Geographical distributions of filovirus outbreaks in Africa, 1997–1999.

a 44-year-old male schoolteacher, became febrile in August 1976 shortly after travelling with six other missionary employees around the far north of Zaire. First treated for malaria, his condition steadily deteriorated, becoming dehydrated with generalised bleeding. He died 1 week later, as did several members of his family. Noticeably his wife survived and she subsequently went on to become an important source of immune plasma. Unbeknown to the missionary sisters, other former patients had also died following their return home. First estimates suggested more than 46 villages were affected with over 350 deaths. Subsequent statistics revealed a case fatality rate in excess of over 90%.

The first report by the Zairian physician Ngoi Mushola was short but accurate—the new affliction was characterised by high temperature, frequent vomiting of black, digested blood, bloody stools and epistaxis. At first sight, these signs resemble yellow fever but this diagnosis was soon discarded when it became known that at least four of the victims had been previously vaccinated. Chest and abdominal pain accompanied by stupor and a state of confusion were common features. But none of these features were familiar to the doctors and missionaries of northern Zaire.

Established in 1935, the sisters in Yambuku had founded a hospital and dispensary in an effort to stem absenteeism in the missionary school. Conditions were basic, exacerbated by an acute shortage of equipment, especially the syringes needed to meet the local expectation that, whatever the ailment, an injection would be forthcoming. Just five syringes were made to last for over 300 patients each day, many being given various combinations of antibiotics, quinine and vitamins. Almost half of the total caseload recorded in this epidemic is likely to have contracted Ebola through the continual reuse of syringes.[3] A fictional account of these events is to be found in the popular book "Ebola", by Close (1995).

During the two 1976 epidemics, the attack rate in infected communities varied from 3.5 to 15.2 per 1000 in the Sudan, and from 8 per 1000 in the centre of the epidemic in Zaire. The attack rate was less, at 1 per 1000, in bordering communities. These findings indicated that the virus was not as highly transmissible as was first feared. Both in the Sudan and in Zaire there was serological evidence of small numbers of minor or even subclinical infections. The secondary attack rate was between 13 and 15% in both countries. The epidemics were readily controlled by isolating the patients and instituting strict barrier nursing with gowns, gloves and masks combined with the treatment of patients' excreta with disinfectants such as formaldehyde and hypochlorite.

A second outbreak of Ebola haemorrhagic fever occurred in southern Sudan during August and September 1979, in the same area as the original 1976 outbreak. There were 34 reported cases, of which 22 were fatal. The clinical diagnosis was confirmed by virus isolation and serology.

The mechanism of transmission of infection in the outbreaks was mainly by direct contact with infected blood, close and prolonged contact with an infected patient,

---

[3] The re-use of syringes continues to be a major source of nosocomial infections in the developing world: WHO estimates that over two million new cases of blood-borne diseases such as HIV, HCV and hepatitis B are the direct result of re-using or improper sterilisation of needles and other sharp instruments (Kane et al., 1999).

accidental inoculation or through the use of contaminated syringes and needles. There was no evidence to suggest respiratory spread in the community although the potential risk of aerosol transmission has been the subject of intense debate. All the major African outbreaks have been characterised by spread within hospitals.

A sporadic case was reported in 1977 in Zaire, 325 km west of the centre of the first outbreak (Heymann et al., 1980). A 9-year-old girl was admitted to the Tandala Mission Hospital with a 3-day history of fever, abdominal pain and haematemesis; she died 1 day later. This case is interesting in that the virus was isolated by inoculation of blood into guinea pigs even after shipment to the USA under less than ideal conditions. This case also stimulated a retrospective study of Ebola virus activity in this locality. Another case was a 45-year-old male who had died some months previously after hospitalisation with a clinical diagnosis of yellow fever. A physician was also found to have been infected; he had a history of a febrile illness in 1972 following accidental injury while performing an autopsy on a patient who was also diagnosed as a case of yellow fever. A 7% seroprevalence of Ebola virus antibodies was found among the local population.

After a gap of over 10 years, the mid-1990s saw a number of outbreaks in Central and West Africa. In early 1995, a charcoal-maker from near Kikwit in eastern Zaire became the first recognised case of an outbreak that over the ensuing 6 months resulted in 315 cases, 77% of which were fatal. The index case transmitted the virus to at least 12 family members. One contact was hospitalised, this admission triggering a series of nosocomial transmissions. Shortly afterwards, a resuscitation team became infected after treating a patient misdiagnosed as having typhoid. The outbreak was inflamed further by the combination of infection of unprotected health personnel and infected patients being returned into the community. As previously in Sudan and Zaire, the situation was brought under control by the application of barrier nursing techniques, disinfection and proper burial of the deceased. Once again, however, the failure of local health authorities to recognise the potential problem and to act swiftly led to a severe hospital-focused outbreak. As previously the rapid introduction of barrier nursing and containment procedures quickly brought this outbreak under control. However, experts returning to Kikwit have noted a return of the more lax standards prevailing before the 1995 outbreak as the memory of its impact recedes, reinforced by a chronic shortage of medical supplies.

Ebola virus has also been found in West Africa within the last decade. A female ethnologist became infected when conducting a post-mortem examination on a chimpanzee found dead in the Tai National Park, Côte d'Ivoire. This case was only diagnosed retrospectively after repatriation to Switzerland but is one of the most complete clinical descriptions (Formenty et al., 1999). Since 1994, three apparently independent outbreaks have occurred in Gabon. In July 1996, the largest of these accounted for over 40 deaths; one patient was treated in South Africa where a fatal nosocomial infection occurred in a nurse.

Ebola virus infection is clearly endemic in northern Congo. Between 4 and 10% of individuals in the Tandala area were found to be antibody-positive by immunofluorescence. Similar evidence of virus infection has been recorded in other savannah regions of Central and West Africa. Antibodies to both filoviruses have been found in 1–2% of selected populations in Nigeria, up to 10% among pygmies and farmers in the rain forest of the Cameroons and 13% in central Liberia. As with the arenaviruses (See Arenaviruses), it is likely that severe haemorrhagic fever may represent an unusual human response to these viruses. Cases appear to be most often misdiagnosed as yellow fever. The case fatality rate is greatest in the early days and weeks of an outbreak, subsequently declining as the causative agent becomes better diagnosed and supportive therapy offered to the patient that much earlier. The risk of transmission increases, however, as the disease progresses owing to higher levels of virus secretion (Dowell et al., 1999).

Johnson et al. (1983) undertook surveillance for Ebola virus infections following two cases of Marburg infection in the west of Kenya in 1980. Evidence of human Ebola infection was uncovered in two schoolgirls from the densely populated Mount Elgon region. Serological evidence of infection was also found in a number of contacts. To the team's surprise, no evidence of Marburg virus infection was found among the 52 suspected cases of acute viral haemorrhagic fever identified in the 21-month-study period. A follow-on study 4 years later between May 1984 and 1985 revealed that nearly 10% of 471 patients with suspected viral haemorrhagic fever had demonstrable antibodies to Ebola virus; the case fatality rate was 5%, no higher than that in those without any evidence of infection. This study also suggested that the virus responsible for these seroconversions belonged to neither of the known serotypes despite cross-reacting with the standard reference strains of Ebola virus.

Unexpectedly, Ebola virus was found during an outbreak of a respiratory disease among macaque monkeys (*M. fascicularis*) housed in a commercial quarantine facility in Reston, Virginia. Within 3 years, a similar outbreak occurred in Siena, Italy. The disease showed the clinical signs and pathological lesions typical of Ebola, with the additional feature of large quantities of virus in respiratory secretions. Despite the high titre of virus present (7×10^6 pfu/ml), there were, fortunately, no cases of human illness among handlers and staff despite occasional evidence of seroconversion. As these animals originated in the Philippines, the outbreak due to the Reston subtype of Ebola may indicate a non-human primate reservoir exists also in Asia. Extensive follow-up studies in the Philippines have not been revealing despite serological evidence of infection in around 6% of monkey handlers and those working in collection areas.

Is there an animal reservoir?

There is a strong suspicion that filoviruses are zoonoses. Monkeys were originally implicated in the three Marburg outbreaks, but there is a lack of evidence suggesting that primates are among the natural reservoirs of the virus, at least on the African continent. Antibody rates were higher toward the end of the two wet seasons, and were three times higher in males than in females. Whatever the identity of the primary animal reservoir, this implies it is a species that expands rapidly after rainfall.

Expert opinion currently states that monkeys likely to become infected from the same reservoir species from which humans can directly become infected. Transmission between monkeys is known to occur only at low efficiency, and antibody rates in captured non-human primates are considerably less than would be the case if filoviruses were maintained in monkeys over long periods of time. The view is further strengthened by the high susceptibility of experimentally infected monkeys. Were any particular species of monkey acting as a primary reservoir in any one locality, evidence of mortality would be expected among wild monkey populations, as is the case, for example, immediately prior to outbreaks of yellow fever.

After the African Ebola viruses were first identified in 1975, Bruce Johnson and his colleagues led an exhaustive (and exhausting) investigation to determine the likely reservoir of the Sudan outbreak, but without success. Focusing on the cotton factory in Nzara where the index case had worked as a clerk, a large number of small animals were caught in and around the factory as well as in the epidemic areas of the Sudan and Zaire. Blood and tissues were removed for investigation in an attempt to throw some light on the natural reservoir but all samples proved negative. Following this disappointment some 200 monkeys and more than 100 other animals were collected in Zaire between 1976 and 1979. Once more no specimens yielded virus and attempts to find Ebola virus antibodies were unsuccessful. However, 26% of peridomestic guinea pigs in the Tandala region proved antibody-positive but tantalisingly there was a lack of correlation between ownership of positive animals and prevalence of antibody in the households concerned. It appears that the guinea pig is an incidental host unlikely to transmit the virus to humans.

There has always been a suspicion that rodents were involved in maintaining the reservoir of Ebola. The hunt for filoviruses has been revived since the introduction of PCR methods for detecting viral genomes and there is an unconfirmed report of Ebola genomes being recovered from rodents trapped in the Central African Republic by scientists from the Pasteur Institute (Morvan et al., 1999). Among 242 animals caught there was evidence of infection in eight using PCR. No infectious virus was recovered from any of the samples. The amplified DNA products bore a close similarity with human Ebola isolates from central Africa (Zaire/Gabon serotype). This was coincidental with the finding of filovirus antibodies to both Ebola and Marburg viruses within the populations of the rain forest, especially among Pigmy groups where the prevalence of antibodies to Ebola virus exceeded 7% (Gonzalez et al., 2000).

The issue of a reservoir for Ebola virus is confounded by the distinct nature of the four virus subtypes that are known to exist, three of which are found in the sub-Saharan region of Africa. The extent of phylogenetic divergence is compatible with the notion that each may have different animal reservoirs, as for example, is the case among arenaviruses and hantaviruses. Thus, in any one geographical locality, there are likely to be different risk profiles for the local inhabitants determined by the habitat and behavioural preferences of the reservoir species.

Monath (1999) has argued that bats may play a role in the transmission cycle, perhaps by predating on insects and arachnids representing the primary hosts. This hypothesis has some attractions. Two of the rare cases of Marburg virus had both visited Kitcum cave near Mount Elgon in East Africa, and bats generally have become increasingly captured as a food source. Many Ebola outbreaks have followed periods of heavy rain which in turn would lead to an escalation in the reproductive behaviour of any arthropod reservoir. A further attraction to the hypothesis is that humans may encounter filoviruses either through a food source, by insect or spider bite, or indirectly by coming into contact with a contaminated environment. It also fits with the evidence that the 1975 case of Marburg virus infection was most likely bitten by an arachnid.

Recent years have seen more evidence of outbreaks coinciding with exposure to non-human primates. Chimpanzees in particular would be at high risk of acquiring infection as they are omnivorous and range from the forest floor to the very top of the forest canopy. Monath (1999) has postulated also that there is frequent contact between humans and non-pathogenic Ebola viruses, if the evidence of serological surveys in Africa is to be believed. This implies sporadic outbreaks occur by favouring pathogenic quasispecies of viral RNA under certain climatic and/or cyclical changes in the numbers of primary and intermediate hosts.

Whatever the nature of the animal reservoirs, the number of recorded outbreaks of Ebola virus has steadily increased in the last decade. It is tempting to assume the numbers reflect increasing awareness on the part of physicians and local public health officials, but this is unlikely to be the sole factor. Outbreaks such as that in Kikwit in 1995 and subsequent outbreaks both in central Africa and in Gabon almost certainly would have been alerted to the international community. More likely is the continuing change in ecological factors combined with the ever increasingly fragile economic infrastructure of the endemic regions. These can readily be seen as tipping the balance in favour of increasing the risk to individuals in communities at forest margins who depend upon subsistence farming. Curiously these outbreaks are invariably attributed to Ebola virus: Marburg virus continues to take a back seat, but this may reflect a less marked effect of environmental changes on the theoretical reservoir of Marburg virus rather than any inherent propensity to be less pathogenic or less virulent.

Morphology and ultrastructure of infected cells

The virions of Ebola and Marburg are similar in morphology to rhabdoviruses, but extensive in length. Marburg and Ebola particles are seen in a variety of forms; these are generally long filaments, sometimes with extensive branching, or as U-shaped, 6-shaped or circular structures (Ellis et al., 1979). Their appearance is so distinctive and aesthetically interesting that micrographs have been hung in art galleries! The particles vary greatly in length (up to 14,000 nm), but have a uniform diameter of 80 nm and an outer membrane covered with 15 nm glycoprotein projections spaced 10 nm apart (Fig. 2). Though the length of Marburg and Ebola particles varies widely, the unit length associated with peak infectivity of Marburg virus is 790 nm. Ebola virus is some 1.2 times longer at 970 nm.

Beneath the virion envelope lies a complex, 20 nm diameter nucleocapsid consisting of a hollow 10–15 nm core surrounded by a helical, tubular capsid of approximately 50 nm; the latter bears cross-striations with a periodicity of about 5 nm. The nucleocapsid structures with a density of 1.32 g/cm^2 can be released from virions by detergent treatment. Structures seen within infected cells are presumed to be virion nucleocapsids because their diameters are close to those of the tubular structures found in intracellular inclusions (Ellis et al., 1978). These bodies are complex and distinct, consisting of a finely

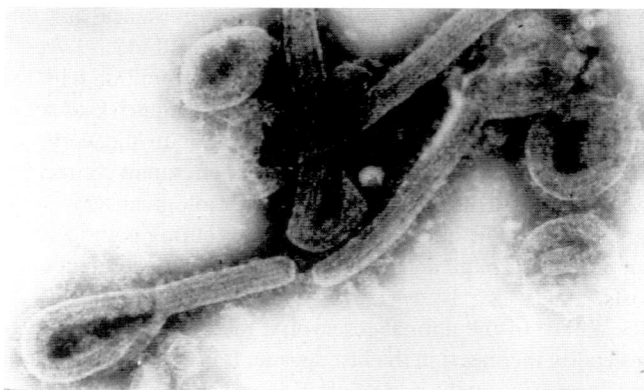

Fig. 2 Negative staining electron microscopy of (a) Marburg and (b) Ebola viruses (micrographs courtesy of Dr D.S. Ellis).

fibrillar or granular ground substance which condenses into either tubular structures or nucleocapsids.

Virions are constructed from preformed nucleocapsids synthesised in the cytoplasm and envelopes are added by budding through cellular membranes. As infection proceeds, these increase in size become highly structured even at sites remote from the cell membranes. The budding of completed virions takes place at cell membranes, into which glycoprotein spikes have been inserted. At the time of maturation from the cell surface a series of individual nucleocapsids becomes enclosed within a single continuous envelope; each individual nucleocapsid is only about 700 nm long when produced in the infected cell. It appears that nucleocapsids, at the time of budding, may orientate relative to the cell membrane, in any plane from perpendicular to parallel, and may undergo the branching characteristic of these viruses. Recent work points to the key role of the VP40 protein, nascent virus particles being inserted into lipid rafts within the plasma membrane. The final infective particle is believed to be the torus form, generated by the flexing of individual core length fragments into a circle or torus.

Physicochemical properties

The extraordinary length of filoviruses makes purification difficult; with an estimated molecular weight in excess of 500×10^6, particles migrate in density gradients very slowly at a sedimentation coefficient of around 1400S equivalent to a molecular mass of approximately $3-6 \times 10^8$. Filoviruses have a buoyant density of 1.14 g/cm^3 in potassium tartrate gradients, which reflect the lipid-containing nature of the outer envelope. Lipid solvents destroy viral infectivity and release the inner nucleocapsid with a density of 1.34 g/cm^3. This ribonucleoprotein complex contains the genome, the major nucleocapsid structural protein (NP) and smaller quantities of other proteins necessary for expression and replication.

In the interest of safety in handling these viruses, knowledge of virion susceptibility to inactivation is important. Infectivity is stable at room temperature but destroyed at 60°C for 30 min. Heating for 60 min adds an extra margin of safety as there are slight differences in the inactivation rates of Ebola and Marburg viruses (Mitchell and McCormick, 1984); this procedure still permits the assay of serum electrolytes, glucose and blood urea in blood samples. The viruses are also inactivated by a variety of physical and chemical treatments, e.g. UV and gamma irradiation, 1% formalin and β-propiolactone. Dilution of blood samples into 3% acetic acid is sufficient to inactivate virus without affecting white blood cell counts (Mitchell and McCormick, 1984). Filoviruses are also inactivated by exposure to various phenolic disinfectants.

Nucleic acid

These are the largest non-segmented negative strand RNA genomes discovered to date. The filoviruses contain a single molecule of RNA with a molecular weight of c. 4.2×10^6 (19.1 kb) rich in uracil and adenosine. The genome is not infectious *per se* and does not contain significant lengths of poly(A) at its $3'$ end, features characteristic of those viral genomes unable to act as viral mRNA without prior RNA polymerase activity. The filoviruses are therefore considered to be negative sense viruses with a strategy of replication and expression broadly similar to that of the rhabdoviruses and paramyxoviruses.

Complete genome sequences are available for Marburg, Ebola and Reston viruses.[4] Both contain seven linearly-arranged genes organised in a similar manner to those of the rhabdoviruses and paramyxoviruses (Fig. 3). The function of these gene products is summarised in Table 2. A unique feature is the presence of both short, overlapping regions between the transcription start sequences and the termination stop site of the upstream gene and intergenic non-coding regions of variable length. The genes are flanked at $3'$ and $5'$ ends by sequences required for transcription and termination, respectively. These are highly conserved among the filoviruses and are characterised by the presence of the hexamer $3'$-UAAUU-$5'$. There is conservation of base sequences at the $3'$ end of both Ebola and Marburg viruses.

Recent estimates of evolutionary divergence suggest that Marburg and Ebola viruses have a substitution rate of 3.6×10^{-5} per nucleotide per year, many hundreds of times less than, e.g. influenza A virus and retroviruses. Thus, Marburg and Ebola diverged at least several thousand years ago (Suzuki and Gojobori, 1997), a divergence that may go some way in explaining the very different frequency with which these two viral species cause outbreaks as each has probably adapted to a distinct animal or insect reservoir occupying ecological niches offering different evolutionary pressures.

---

[4] Reference numbers NC 001608 (Marburg), NC002549 (Zaire) and NC 004161 (Reston) on the NCBI website (http://www.ncbi.nlm.nih.gov).

144

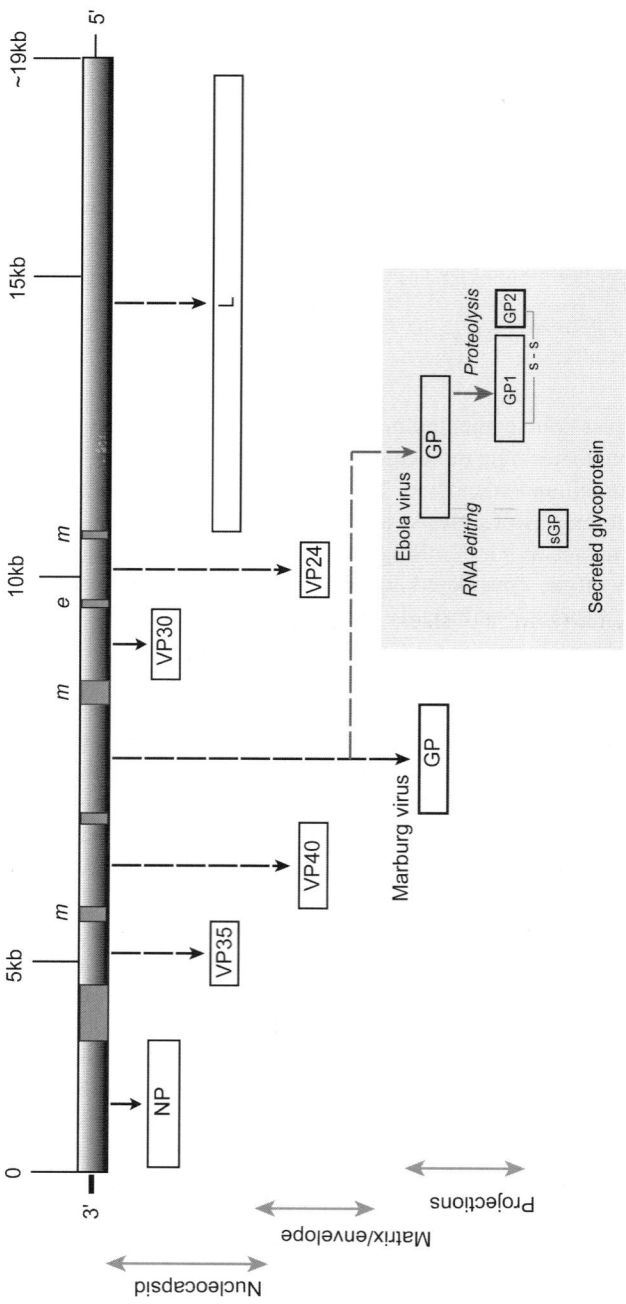

Fig. 3 Genetic organisation of the filovirus genome.

Table 2

Filovirus gene products

Protein	Size (molecular weight)[a]	Function
NP	78 kb	Major nucleocapsid structural protein
VP35	31 kb	Bound to nucleocapsid: RNA polymerase modulator
VP40	32 kb	Matrix structural protein
GP	75 kb (170 kb)[b]	Envelope glycoprotein
sGP [Ebola]	15 kb	Secreted glycoprotein: modulates host immune response?
VP30	32 kb	Minor nucleocapsid protein
VP24	29 kb	Matrix or membrane associated
L	267 kb	RNA polymerase: transcriptional replication

[a]Estimates from cloned genes of Marburg virus.
[b]Estimates of glycosylated form resolved by SDS-PAGE.

Proteins

Both Ebola and Marburg viruses contain seven major polypeptides expressed monocistronically (Fig. 3). In many respects the assignment of proteins to structural components closely resembles that of the rhabdoviruses, a finding that at first prompted attempts to classify both agents within the Rhabdoviridae. However, there are important differences, particularly in the sizes of the major virion polypeptides and in the expression of the glycoprotein gene. Ebola virus consists of an internal nucleocapsid with one major polypeptide (NP) of molecular weight 78,000, the outer envelope with a single glycoprotein (GP) of molecular weight 170,000 and a further large protein (L) of molecular weight 267,000. Additionally, there are four other structural proteins, VP40, VP35, VP30 and VP24, so designated after their respective molecular weights (Elliott et al., 1985). VP24 is found within the matrix but is less abundant than VP40. Detergent treatment of purified virions releases the viral nucleocapsid: the VP35 remains bound under low salt conditions, suggesting that this polypeptide may have a functional role similar to that of the P protein of paramyxoviruses and rhabdoviruses. The fourth nucleocapsid protein (VP30) is required for transcription (Muhlberger et al., 1999).

The VP40 protein is the most abundant, being a matrix protein similar to that of other enveloped, negative-strand RNA viruses. VP40 consists of two domains with unique folds, linked by a flexible dimer. X-ray crystallography suggests a model whereby hexamers are created by aggregation of the N-terminal sequence: the C-terminus mediates lipid binding. A conformational change leading to hexamerisation may therefore be an important step in virus assembly (Dessen et al., 2000; Ruigrok et al., 2000). It is unique amongst viral matrix proteins in containing two overlapping domains (L-domains) that recognise cellular proteins during the process of maturation and budding.

Less is known regarding VP24, but a role in virulence is suggested by the finding that Ebola virus variants adapted to growth in guinea pigs showed a mutation at either amino acid 186 or 187 (histidine to tyrosine, and threonine to isoleucine, respectively).

Insertions and deletions at the GP editing site appear to affect both transcription and genome replication (Volchkov et al., 2000).

As GP1 is the only distal surface protein, it is likely to bear cellular receptors as it mediates infection by VSV as well as retrovirus pseudotypes. The glycoproteins of Marburg and the four subtypes of Ebola differ markedly in terms of gene expression. The glycoprotein gene of Marburg is expressed as a single gene product whereas the Ebola genome codes for the two glycoproteins in two reading frames; the products are expressed as a result of transcriptional editing and translational frame shifting (Feldmann et al., 1994). The Ebola virus structural glycoprotein (GP) forms the envelope peplomers; the second glycoprotein of molecular weight 15,000 (sGP) is made in considerable quantities and secreted as soluble protein from the infected cell (Sanchez et al., 1998).

Viral proteins are frequently synthesised in a non-active form in order that assembly and viral release can progress unhindered. The glycoproteins of filoviruses are initially expressed as single chain precursors that are immediately transferred to the endoplasmic reticulum for post-translational cleavage and glycosylation. Post-translational cleavage then generates two functional products, GP1 and GP2 in a manner analogous to the creation of the HA1 and HA2 haemagglutinin components of influenza virus and to the generation of the gp120 and gp41 structural proteins of HIV. This analogy is an important one as it suggests cleavage is an essential prerequisite for activating the function of the glycoproteins, in particular a membrane fusion property essential for the next round of virus replication. The glycoprotein GP2 of Ebola virus spontaneously forms a trimeric, α-helical, rod-shaped structure (Weissenhorn et al., 1998; Malashkevich et al., 1999). This coiled—coil structure of GP2 is comparable with the structure seen of other viral glycoproteins known to play a role in membrane fusion.

The filovirus GP precursor is cleaved by the protein convertase furin, a protease ubiquitous on the surface of mammalian cells and is particularly rich on the surfaces of liver hepatocytes and endothelial cells, two key cellular targets for filoviruses. This picture is not too dissimilar to the situation for myxoviruses, where such protein convertases are responsible for systemic spread (Klenk and Rott, 1988). Furin is a processing enzyme of the constitutive secretory pathway of mammalian cells, being one of a number of enzymes that recognise basic sequence motifs such as R-x-K/R-R, where x may be any amino acid. This cleavage is essential for virus activation and full infectivity in the next round of virus replication. This event is expected to trigger a conformational change and exposure of a domain on GP necessary for fusion with cellular membranes during virus entry (Feldmann et al., 2003).

Processing of glycoproteins is likely to confer virulence as suggested by the observation that the Reston strain, considered as not pathogenic for humans (Fisher-Hoch et al., 1992) has the motif K-Q-K/R-R, not the optimal sequence motif for recognition by fucin. Fucin-mediated cleavage can be inhibited by peptidyl chloromethylketones, thus offering the possible route for developing a specific antiviral inhibitor (Anderson et al., 1993).

Variation among isolates

Phylogenetic analyses clearly show Marburg and Ebola as distinct viruses, and that each of the four Ebola virus antigens is sufficiently distinctive as to suggest differences in virus–host relationships. This has profound implications for understanding filovirus epidemiology, as each may have its own host reservoir and pathogenic properties. The difference among Ebola isolates is often substantial, with sequence variability being as great at 47%. Interestingly, the monkey-associated Reston subtype shows a closer identity with the Sudan subtype than with the cluster of Ebola isolates from Zaire and Gabon (Georges-Courbot et al., 1997).

Genome sequencing has shown subsequently that isolates obtained at different times, either within Sudan or Zaire, are of similar genotype but are distinguishable from those taken from patients at any other locality.

Two Zaire strains isolated a year apart were found to be genotypically identical and a similar analysis of five isolates from the Sudan over a 3 year period showed only a limited change. This finding illustrates that Ebola virus is genetically stable to the same degree as other members of the order Mononegavirales. This has been illustrated dramatically by the finding of high genetic homology between the 1976 Zaire strains with those causing the Kikwit outbreak 19 years later.

The differences between the two African Ebola virus strains from Sudan and Zaire are reflected in their antigenic properties. Sera from immune individuals contain substantially higher titres of antibodies against the homologous than against the heterologous virus; this reaction appears asymmetric, as sera from patients in Zaire react better with the Sudan virus than vice versa. Absorption of human antisera with heterologous virus enhances the specificity of these reactions; Richman et al. (1983) reported that absorption of antiserum to a Zaire strain with the "Boniface" isolate from Sudan reduced binding to the homologous antigen by over 40%, whereas binding to Boniface antigens was completely abolished.

Replication

For many years, research on filovirus replication was severely hampered by the issues surrounding the safe handling of these viruses. The situation has now changed since the DNA cloning of filovirus RNA and progress is now rapidly being made using *in vitro* expression systems.

Much is now being discovered as to the intracellular events accompanying filovirus replication. Elliott et al. (1985) examined viral protein synthesis in Ebola-infected cells by means of immunoprecipitation, as host cell protein synthesis is not inhibited significantly by virus growth. Strains from the Sudan appeared to have a longer growth cycle than virus from Zaire. Both the nucleocapsid protein (NP) and the major envelope glycoprotein (GP) could be detected by 6 h after infection. Viral mRNA was first detected at 7 h, reached a peak by 18 h and thereafter declined (Sanchez and Kiley, 1987). A total of six monocistronic mRNAs has been detected but so far virion RNA has not been found within infected cells.

Resolution of virus-specific polypeptides is helped by the addition of actinomycin D to reduce the level of host gene transcription. The most abundant protein, the membrane-associated protein VP40, appears at 12 h, later than the appearance of VP35 at 8 h, which implies a regulatory role for this minor virus component. The nucleocapsid NP and VP30 proteins are phosphorylated during the growth cycle, possibly as part of a mechanism that controls expression and replication of the genome in ribonucleoprotein complexes, but this is speculative.

The extraordinary high numbers of virus particles released from infected cells implies an efficient mechanism of assembly and maturation. Nascent Ebola virus buds from lipid rafts embedded in the cellular plasma membrane (Bavari et al., 2002).

Diagnosis

Virus is readily isolated from blood or serum using Vero E6 cells. Virus can also be isolated from other body fluids, e.g. semen and throat washings. Filoviruses do not normally cause an extensive cytopathic effect; however, and thus the developing cytoplasmic inclusion bodies are best detected by addition of specific antibodies to fixed cells. A positive diagnosis is usually forthcoming from 3 to 5 days after inoculation of cell cultures. Some difficulty arose with isolating the Sudanese strains of Ebola in cell culture, however, and intraperitoneal inoculation of guinea pigs has in the past been necessary in order to amplify the virus prior to detection by cell culture.

Electron microscopy remains a useful diagnostic tool, as was shown in controlling the Reston outbreak (Geisbert and Jahrling, 1990). Although the morphology of filoviruses is unmistakable, it is less easy to differentiate between different filoviruses by this method unless immune electron microscopy is employed.

Immunofluorescence for the detection of antibodies (IFA) is the test of choice: infected Vero cells are readily prepared, inactivated and shipped to field laboratories (Rollin et al., 1990). The presence of IgM antibodies together with clinical symptoms of haemorrhagic disease is usually sufficient for a confirmed diagnosis. Paired samples are necessary for diagnosis if reliance is placed on detecting IgG antibodies, with a greater than 64-fold rise indicative of acute filovirus infection. In the last few years, baculovirus-expressed nucleocapsid protein has become available, thus opening up alternative diagnostic technologies.

During the Kikwit outbreak in Zaire, an antigen capture solid phase immunoassay was used with some success. Plates coated with monoclonal antibody were used to capture viral antigens in serum and bound antigen detected using rabbit polyclonal antiserum (Ksiazek et al., 1992). Also during this outbreak it was found that skin biopsies contain considerable amounts of viral antigen, thus offering an alternative method for confirming diagnoses (Zaki et al., 1999).

Further advances have seen the development of an assay for detecting antibodies directed against a conserved, immunodominant epitope on the nucleocapsid protein has been described by Meissner et al. (2002). These authors isolated a human monoclonal antibody against the Zaire strain from a donor convalescent from the 1995 outbreak in Kikwit. The antigen-combining Fab fragment of this antibody was cloned into phagemid

DNA and phage produced in *Escherichia coli* (Maruyama et al., 1999a,b). Binding was visualised by prestaining of the fab-phage particles with Disperse Red dye. Antibody was successfully detected in all 10 convalescent sera examined by competition inhibition.

Clinical features

Filovirus infections of humans are characterised by a sudden onset, a high case fatality ratio, and significant potential for person to person transmission. The pathology of the disease is similar in both humans and non-human primates, and thus monkeys have been intensively studied as models of filovirus disease. The pathological picture is one of extensive involvement of the liver and kidneys, accompanied by changes in vascular permeability, endothelial damage and activation of the clotting cascade. The critical question, however, is what actually causes death as the extensive necrosis of soft tissue resulting from virus replication is not alone responsible for the high mortality.

There is strong evidence to implicate filovirus replication in macrophages and monocytes in the key early stages of disease progression. Post-mortem studies have shown that endothelial cells become heavily involved in the acute phase, and the lysis that results destroys endothelial function.

Evidence also exists for active mediators enhancing the disease process. Feldman et al. (1996), for example, have shown that the supernatants of macrophage cultures infected with Marburg virus increases paraendothelial permeability. Elevated levels of secreted cytokines such as TNF-α may therefore be instrumental in initiating the shock syndrome seen in severe and fatal cases. The resulting loss of endothelial integrity that develops as a consequence augments further rounds of virus growth, ending in vascular permeability and the triggering of the coagulation process.

The illnesses caused in man by Marburg and Ebola viruses are virtually indistinguishable. The incubation period was 3–9 days in both the early German and South African outbreaks of Marburg disease, but in the later Ebola epidemics a wider range of 4–16 days is more often the norm. Both infections have abrupt onset with frontal and temporal headaches, followed by high fever and generalised pains, particularly in the back. A relative bradycardia is frequently an early sign. Patients rapidly become prostrated and some develop severe watery diarrhoea leading to rapid dehydration and weight loss. Diarrhoea, abdominal pain with cramping nausea, and vomiting may persist for a week. In the 1977 Sudanese outbreak, knife-like chest and pleuritic pain was an early symptom and many patients complained of a very dry, rather than sore, throat accompanied by a cough. In the Sudanese Ebola outbreak, pharyngitis was commonly noted, accompanied by fissuring with open sores on the tongue and lips.

On white skin, a characteristic non-itching maculopapular rash appeared between days 5 and 7, lasting 3–4 days. This was followed by a fine desquamation. On pigmented skin, the rash, often described as measles-like, is not so obvious and is often recognised only during desquamation.

Conjunctivitis has been a consistent feature in all cases. An enanthem of the palate was reported in the Marburg outbreak in Germany, but not in the three South African cases. Irritation and inflammation of the scrotum or labia majora were common, with orchitis occurring in a few patients. Pancreatitis has been noted in several cases.

Patients with Ebola virus infection admitted to hospital at the onset of illness frequently give the appearance of being 'ghost-like'; they appear withdrawn with anxious features, expressionless faces, deep-set eyes and a greyish pallor. All patients are extremely lethargic (Fig. 4). Involvement of the central nervous system infections has been apparent in a number of cases, with signs of meningeal irritation, paraesthesia, lethargy, confusion, irritability and aggression.

Many patients in both the Marburg and the Ebola outbreaks developed severe bleeding between days 5 and 7. The gastrointestinal tract and lungs were most often affected, with haematemesis, malaena and sometimes the passage of fresh blood in the stools. There was also bleeding from the nose, gums and vagina; subconjunctival

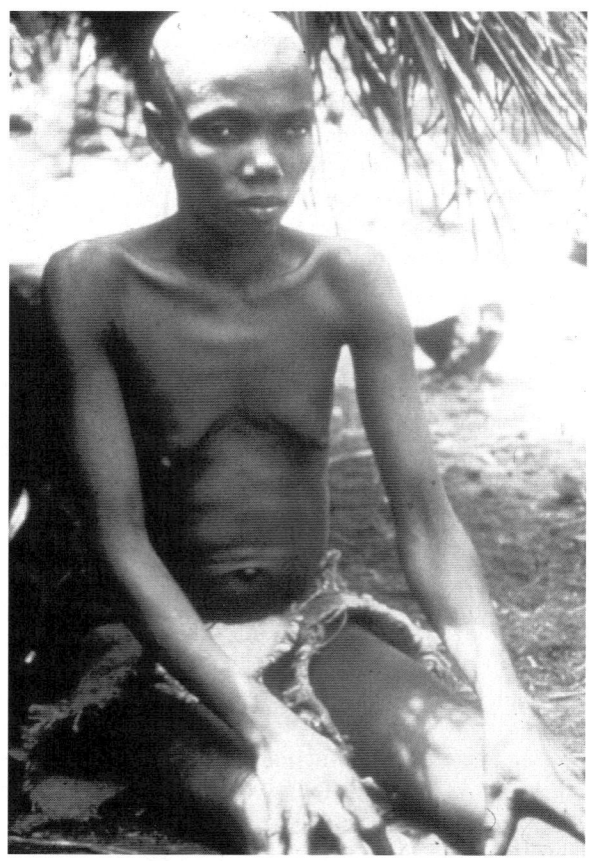

Fig. 4 Patient with Ebola virus, Sudan, 1977, showing the typical withdrawn facial features and emaciated appearance (photograph courtesy of Professor David Simpson).

haemorrhages were common, as were petechiae and bleeding from needle puncture sites. Laboratory investigations of the early Marburg-related outbreaks suggested that in some patients there was disseminated intravascular coagulation with subsequent kidney failure. Leucopenia early in the course of illness is a constant feature, followed by leucocytosis and a low erythrocyte sedimentation rate. The acquired Pelger–Huet anomaly of the neutrophils and atypical mononuclear cells have been observed. Thrombocytopenia is recorded in most patients from about day 3 onwards.

Death generally occurs between days 6 and 9 after the onset of clinical disease and is usually preceded by severe blood loss and shock. In surviving patients, recovery is slow and debilitating, frequently accompanied by amnesia, which may persist for many weeks. Abortion is common among pregnant women and the infants born to mothers in the terminal stage of the disease are invariably infected.

It is a feature of filovirus infections that there is no evidence of appreciable virus shedding by any route other than that of haemorrhage. Substantive evidence of aerosol transmission is lacking, with very little virus being found in the throat or urine. However, the persistence of virus in some body fluids up to 83 days after onset does pose a risk of late transmission. One of the South African Marburg patients developed uveitis 2 months after recovery, with virus successfully cultured from fluid aspirated from the anterior chamber. Experience in the 1995 Kikwit outbreak showed that the skin may also harbour virus. Thus, the mere touching of an infected person may facilitate the virus to spread.

Isolation of patients, rigorous adherence to aseptic techniques and the adoption of precautions for enteric type diseases are a minimum for adequate biological containment of these viruses. Strict barrier nursing conditions are an absolute must, with personnel using a double gown complete with an impervious lining, double gloves and a respirator, preferably fitted with a HEPA filter. The handling of specimens for virus serology and isolation requires Biosafety Level 4 facilities.

The effectiveness of such precautions was aptly demonstrated during the Kikwit outbreak of 1995. A total of 76 medical staff acquired Ebola virus during the first week of the outbreak by direct contact with patients. However, only one case was reported after strict isolation procedures together with barrier nursing procedures were introduced.

Pathology

Filoviruses are pantropic, producing lesions in nearly every organ. However, the most affected are the liver and spleen. Vascular changes include haemorrhages, occlusions and thromboses. At autopsy, swelling of the spleen, lymph nodes and kidney is frequently present. Petechiae are seen in the mucosae of the stomach and small intestine. Haemorrhage occurs into the skin, mucous membranes and gastrointestinal tract, with the stomach and parts of the intestines becoming filled with blood. This makes for the safe care of patients particularly difficult, although there is considerable debate amongst prominent experts as to just how great a risk acutely patients present to those nursing them.

Histological examination of the liver and lymphoid tissue enables a reasonably accurate diagnosis. There is severe degeneration of lymphoid tissue with necrosis in the spleen and liver. Focal hepatic necrosis is accompanied by the formation of eosinophilic bodies—resembling the Councilman bodies of yellow fever—and smaller, basophilic inclusions; both types can also be seen in most other tissues. The fatty changes within hepatocytes, so characteristic of yellow fever, are, however, slight. Mononuclear cells accumulate in the peripheral spaces. Even at the height of the necrotic process in the liver there is evidence of hepatocyte regeneration. High concentrations of virus are seen by electron microscopy in the zones of necrosis.

Necrotic lesions are also found in the pancreas, gonads, adrenals, hypophysis, thyroid, kidney and skin. Severe congestion and stasis are obvious in the spleen. There are few lesions in the lungs except for circumscribed haemorrhages and endarteritis, especially of arterioles. Neuropathological changes are confined mainly to the glial elements throughout the brain. Congestion of meningeal and intracerebral blood vessels has been observed in the brains of experimentally infected rhesus monkeys, possibly indicating early thrombosis and consistent with the confused behaviour and other neurological signs in many patients with Ebola virus infection.

Acute Ebola virus infection in rhesus monkeys closely resembles the illness in man, producing considerable insight as to just how the filoviruses result in haemorrhage and shock. The importance of widespread injury to small blood vessels and capillaries in all organs has become clear from sequential studies (Baskerville et al., 1985). The endothelial necrosis accompanying virus replication leads to the separation of junctions between epithelial cells and detachment from basement membranes. In turn, these focal lesions result in haemorrhage and oedema. Defective platelet aggregation precedes a fall in the platelet count. The prolongation of coagulation times suggests a defect in prostacyclin production. The late stages of the disease are accompanied by extensive intravascular fibrin deposition and an increase in fibrin degradation products. The end result is a generalised loss of epithelial integrity leading to the rapid onset of haemorrhage and shock.

The profound leucopenia may result from the neutrophil inactivation by soluble glycoprotein secreted from virus infected cells. It has been postulated that this is mediated by CD16 molecules which are exclusively found on neutrophils and represent the IgG Fc receptor IIIb (Yang et al., 1998). This is paralleled by virus infection of mononuclear phagocytes and the fibroblastic reticular system, thereby disrupting antigen processing and excessive cytokine production. This in turn accelerates further liver damage. The major envelope glycoprotein GP possesses a possible immunosuppression motif which may also contribute to the host's failure to mount an effected immune response (Volchkov et al., 1992). There is evidence that GP2 binding to epithelial cells is sufficient to trigger the haemorrhagic manifestation of the disease through a process of vascular instability and shock.

Treatment and prevention

At present there is no specific treatment for filovirus infections. The anticipation of complications such as shock, cerebral oedema, renal failure and hypertension can do much to improve management and supportive care is essential. Anticoagulant therapy has been used for two patients with Marburg infection (Gear et al., 1975), although the use of heparin remains controversial.

On November 5, 1976 a scientist working at Porton Down punctured a thumb whilst attempting to passage virus between guinea pigs. Although no blood was drawn, he developed a febrile illness within a week. Virus was abundantly seen in his blood by electron microscopy. Placed inside a negative pressure isolator, the next weeks saw his condition deteriorate, with symptoms in common with African victims of Ebola. Unlike those in Africa, however, the patient could be intensively nursed and electrolyte balance maintained. He was also treated with human β-lymphoblastoid interferon twice a day from a preparation originally allocated for a study of chronic hepatitis B in London's Kings College. Within 2 days after onset, he also received immune plasma from Sophie, the surviving wife of the index case in Yambuku. Viraemia decreased by over 4 logs soon after transfusion, and 7 days later virus could not be isolated. After 9 days, his situation improved and he was discharged nearly 50 days after being isolated. Whether the interferon or the immune plasma was responsible for his improvement is hard to say. Certainly immune plasma has been used to great effect in treating patients with Junin (see Arenaviruses) but there is only limited evidence showing that convalescent human serum can neutralise Ebola virus infectivity (Maruyama et al., 199b). Passive transfer of antibody to monkeys has not been found to give long term protection (Jahrling et al., 1999).

Passive immunisation

During the 1976 Ebola outbreak in northern Congo, several missionary staff were evacuated to Kinshasa for treatment. At this point, the belief was that the epidemic was due to Marburg. Thus, the experience of Dr Isaacson was called upon who had treated two Australian backpackers the previous year in South Africa. A student nurse, Mayinga N'Saka, who became infected caring for the Catholic sisters in Kinshasa's Ngalieme Hospital was given two doses of Marburg immune plasma, but to little effect. A blood sample from this nurse produced the Mayinga strain of Ebola virus.

Convalescent sera were administered during the Kikwit outbreak of Ebola virus but firm conclusions are difficult to draw as there was the inevitable lack of controls (Mupapa et al., 1999). The key role of the envelope glycoprotein has led to the suggestion that anti-glycoprotein antibodies may have some value in post-exposure therapy, but work in the guinea pig and other animals has shown a spectrum of efficacy illustrating this may be more difficult to achieve than was at first thought. Several monoclonal antibodies previously shown to neutralise Marburg virus infectivity *in vitro* proved to offer only partial protection *in vivo* (Hevey et al., 2003). Three murine antibodies against non-overlapping sites on Ebola virus glycoprotein provided protection at most in 60% of the animals challenged with 1000 pfu of virus, despite prior immunisation with a large volume of antibodies in the form of ascites fluid. This contrasts with the findings of Wilson et al. (2000) who showed that mice could be passively protected from challenge with Ebola virus. One complication is that monoclonal antibodies with protective capacity recognise epitopes on the viral glycoprotein outside of the domain bordered by residues 389–493 bearing the neutralising domains of the GP1 molecule (Wilson et al., 2000; Takada et al., 2003). In all probability, the neutralising antibody response is directed against conformational rather than linear epitopes. The limited success in guinea pigs may reflect that conformational specificity is that much more important in neutralising the infectivity of virus for guinea pigs. This is partly borne out by the work of Takada and colleagues who have demonstrated that antigenic variants of Ebola virus selected in the presence of neutralising monoclonal antibodies have amino acid substitutions widely spaced on the linear amino acid sequence of the GP molecule (Takada et al., 2003). The role of carbohydrate side chains in determining the conformation and properties of the glycoprotein is unknown, but may have a considerable bearing as to the immunogenicity of GP1 and the longevity of the response.

Studies using a mouse model have been encouraging. Both passive transfer of antibodies and adoptive transfer of immune cells protected mice against challenge with infectious virus (Gupta et al., 2001; Wilson and Hart, 2001). Ideally antibodies should not be reactive against the soluble form of Ebola virus glycoprotein (sGP) as this form can adsorb neutralising antibodies and is abundantly expressed during the acute phase (Sanchez et al., 1996). In this context, it is worth noting that Wilson and colleagues successfully protected mice from challenge with Ebola virus using monoclonal antibodies recognising only the soluble form of GP (Wilson et al., 2000). There are comparatively few cross-reactive neutralising epitopes between the different strains of Ebola virus (Takada and Kawaoka, 2001), however, and this will further complicate vaccine development. The design of a vaccine capable of inducing additional, cellular immune responses would likely confer a broader vaccine specificity as it is well known with other viruses that epitopes recognised by virus-specific cytotoxic T cells are conserved across virus serotypes.

Active immunisation

No licensed vaccine is available for these diseases, although such a product would be of value for protecting healthcare personnel in Africa and laboratory staff who handle tissues and cells from captured wild monkeys. The development of Ebola vaccines is fraught with difficulties. A strategy of attenuating or inactivating infectious virus is unlikely to be accepted on safety grounds. Moreover, there will have to be a heavy reliance on challenge experiments using experimental animals offering a close simulation of human responses as efficacy studies in man are inconceivable. Such animal work has to be carried out in housing to the highest level of biosafety, compounding the difficulties. If this was not sufficient a disincentive for commercial manufacturers, the limited market size places filovirus vaccines beyond commercial viability, given that any new vaccine product requires a research and development budget in excess of $350 million.

The difficulty has been extending these studies to primates, where protection against disease has been considerably more difficult to reproduce.

Against this background, there have been significant advances in the public sector by taking advantage of DNA clones, recombinant proteins and various vectors. Attempts to formulate a vaccine have focused on stimulating antibodies to the major envelope protein, GP1, as this is known to induce neutralising antibodies. If antibody alone is all that is required for prophylaxis, this is complicated by the fact that neutralising domains are also present on the secreted form (sGP), thus sGP may adsorb neutralising antibodies *in vivo*. This may explain the difficulties in detecting neutralising antibodies in patients' sera.

Several groups have attempted to exploit the property of DNA immunogens to stimulate both class I and class II immune responses. Although DNA immunisation with a plasmid expressing Ebola GP protected guinea pigs against challenge (Xu et al., 1998), these findings have not been reproduced in non-human primates. The most promising are a series of recent studies by Sullivan and her colleagues at the National Institutes of Health and the United States Army Research Institute for Infectious Diseases. Guinea pigs were first injected with DNA encoding for the Ebola virus glycoprotein: the anti-GP antibody response was then boosted with the same viral sequence expressed via an adenovirus 5 vector. Immune animals successfully resisted challenge with a rodent-adapted strain of Ebola (Sullivan et al., 2000). Sufficiently encouraged, Sullivan and colleagues then proceeded to repeat these experiments in a small group of four monkeys. The immunisation process resulted in the complete protection of three animals, the fourth succumbing only to an asymptomatic infection. However, the validity of these findings at this point in the programme was restricted owing to the small challenge dose (six plaque-forming units) used for the challenge.

A "prime-boost" strategy is a further refinement of this approach. Three inoculations of macaque monkeys over 8 weeks with the plasmid containing the GP of the Zaire serotype was followed by a boost at 20 weeks using a disabled adenovirus type 5 vector expressing the homologous viral protein (Sullivan et al., 2003). Virus-specific antibodies were detected by week 12 and all of the animals resisted the virus challenge and survived.

Although encouraging, the prime-boost approach is clearly impractical for field use, particularly when multiple visits would be required to targeted recipients living in remote areas. A recent study by Sullivan et al. (2003) using either one or two doses of the adenovirus vector with the GP protein alone suggests an alternative, much quicker route to protective immunity is possible. Although the titre of anti-GP antibodies was lower, the animals were solidly protected against challenge with live virus. The importance of this observation is that it opens up the concept of a single shot vaccine for diseases like Ebola, although it should be noted that in these studies single dose immunisations were carried out with a mixture of vectors expressing both GP and N proteins. In contrast to earlier studies, the challenge dose at 1500 pfu was considerably higher than that used previously, making this set of experiments much more valid in terms of vaccine development. Also noteworthy was the observed increase in CD8 + cytotoxic lymphocytes (CTLs) in five of eight animals that accompanied the development of immunity. Protection may thus be enhanced after a single dose by the development of both virus-specific antibody and cellular responses.

Attenuated live vectors are attractive as vehicles for stimulating both arms of the immune response. Work towards a filovirus vaccine has also been carried out using a disabled Venezuelan Equine Encephalitis (VEE) virus vector expressing Marburg virus protein. In these experiments, the vaccinated animals withstood a much higher dose of challenge virus. There is clear evidence that glycoprotein expressed as either a recombinant protein or as part of an alphavirus replicon system will protect guinea pigs from challenge with Marburg virus (Hevey et al., 1998). The key issue, however, is whether such vaccines will protect primates: as mentioned above there have been a number of previous studies showing how difficult it is to extend these positive observations to target species.

As with other RNA viruses where vaccines are difficult to design, the use of reverse genetics is likely to precipitate further developments towards a filovirus vaccine. Volchkov et al. (2001) constructed a DNA molecule opposite in polarity to the native Ebola virus genome. By introducing this full-length complementary DNA copy into cells also transfected with DNA coding for Ebola virus genomes, this group successfully produced nascent virus particles that were infectious for fresh cell cultures. This success opens up a myriad of possibilities for altering or modifying determinants of pathogenicity whilst retaining the capacity to stimulate a protective immune response.

All of these studies are constrained conceptually; however, due to a dearth of information as to what type of immune response is required for protection, and what would be the necessary specificity towards the viral proteins. Applying Ebola or Marburg vaccines—once available—may prove to be an even greater task. If these hurdles were to be overcome, there remains the issue of many targeted populations being burdened with a high prevalence of immunosuppressing parasitic diseases and HIV, and thus may not be fully reactive to any vaccine. It is clear that much more needs to be known about the properties of these viruses and the diseases they cause before the development of effective vaccines is realised.

Summary

Of all the viral haemorrhagic fevers the filoviruses present by far the greatest difficulties and challenges. Despite intensive efforts since the Sudan and Zaire outbreaks of 1997, we remain completely ignorant as to the identity of the animal reservoirs for Marburg and Ebola viruses. Without this knowledge, it is hard to see how the epidemiology of filovirus disease can begin to be understood in terms of dynamics and indicators of disease outbreaks. Yet these epidemics are now common in Central Africa and experts in the field

Table 3

Filoviruses—key questions

What are the reservoirs of Marburg and Ebola viruses, and how are these viruses maintained within these animal reservoirs?
What is the mechanism by which filoviruses cause a severe, pantropic infection in humans?
What is the pathological significance of the expression of soluble envelope glycoprotein by Ebola viruses?
Are additional filoviruses awaiting to be discovered on continents other than Africa?
How can the lessons of containment and control be translated into sustainable health policies for those countries most at risk?
How will candidate filovirus vaccines be tested for efficacy?

---

fear such outbreaks will only intensify unless a serious international effort is mounted to understand better the epidemiology of these diseases. A continuing paradox is that Marburg virus appears far less prevalent in Africa than Ebola virus. Only a handful of cases have come to our attention over the past 50 years although serological studies suggest native populations in Central Africa are exposed to this virus on a regular basis. Perhaps Marburg virus has less potential to cause serious human illness or has a more stable relationship with its native animal host, and this is less affected by the pace of environmental change within its endemic area. The only modicum of comfort is that outbreaks can be quickly contained if recognised sufficiently early and strict barrier nursing procedures instituted at once. Unfortunately even this simple lesson is not learnt easily and lapses in standards quickly set in as memory of an outbreak fades. More optimistically, tangible progress is now being made towards the development of candidate Ebola virus vaccines, but how these will be tested—and paid for—is likely to prove as equally challenging as answering the more fundamental scientific questions as to epidemiology and pathology.

Comment and perspectives

New threats to public health are now emerging at the rate of around one per year, with over 30 appearing in the last three decades. Many of these are the consequences of diseases crossing species barriers, especially from wildlife reservoirs and domesticated animals to humans. Diseases and their vectors are adapting to new ecosystems, accelerated by longer term climatic changes resulting from greenhouse gas emissions and forest clearing and the inexorable rise in the global human population. Every populated continent has experienced new diseases, regardless of their economic status. Dengue is an excellent case in point. Prior to 1970, epidemics were restricted to as few as nine countries. Now, a generation later, over 55 countries now see regular outbreaks are at high risk of dengue virus incursion. This has been largely due to the rapid geographical expansion of *Aedes aegypti* following the collapse of insecticide spraying programmes. Rodents as major reservoirs of arenaviruses and hantaviruses have thrived at the expense of other species in regions where there has been substantial changes to the ecosystem, their numbers increasing even further under abnormal climatic conditions. The influence of environmental changes on the behaviour of filoviruses is suspected but with no evidence as to the major reservoirs for Marburg and Ebola, predicting outbreaks of these diseases is all but impossible. In general terms, these observations translate into a need for understanding better ecosystems of those regions in which viral haemorrhagic fevers erupt, otherwise the prediction of outbreaks will remain impossible. That this can be done is shown by studies of vegetation based on satellite imagery leading to the successful prediction of Rift Valley fever outbreaks.

Global surveillance and control

Viral haemorrhagic fevers are among those diseases that impact upon health and the economy of nations. Concern as to the spread of these agents and other emerging diseases has never been greater. As mentioned in 'Introduction', sustained surveillance is the key to effective control. International effort has been strengthened considerably since 2001 with the introduction of a more integrated system of national and international reporting, this being focused as it is in discerning trends and collecting background data. This is a fundamental shift in approach that is being led by international agencies, in particular the World Health Organisation. The difficulty is that outbreaks of new diseases often occur in countries that lack suitable epidemiological expertise, national monitoring laboratories and clinical personnel trained in recognising the unusual and reacting to it in a manner consistent with containing an emerging outbreak. Outbreaks of Ebola and Lassa fevers are particularly centred on regions devoid of this essential infrastructure. These issues have been discussed in depth by Heymann and Rodier (2001).[1]

Concern is now mounting that Rift Valley fever virus could easily spread beyond Africa into heavily populated regions of Europe and elsewhere. There are the first signs of such a spread: an outbreak in Saudi Arabia in 2000 shows just how easily the virus can spread without warning. Mosquito competence, i.e. the inherent ability to amplify the virus, has been shown in the laboratory for a number of mosquito species found in North America and elsewhere in the northern hemisphere.

The high viraemia in susceptible hosts combined with the existence of potential mosquito vectors outside of the present-day confines of the endemic areas of Africa represents a real threat to the global livestock industry. It is simply a matter of time before Rift Valley fever expands outside of Africa, either by inadvertent importation of an infected vector or by a deliberate act of bioterrorism. Soberingly, the USA is now dealing each summer with an increasing number of cases of West Nile fever since the inadvertent introduction of this virus from the Middle East into the New York area in 1999. The cost of this incursion alone is estimated at around $100 m. This incursion illustrates vividly the problems of containing an arthropod-borne pathogen once it has been introduced into a susceptible population of vectors. Importantly, events in 1999 showed how important it is to ensure those responsible for public health liaise fully and openly with animal health and agricultural agencies. Although not a viral disease, bovine spongiform encephalopathy (BSE) in the United Kingdom showed just how technological changes in the animal and food chain can impact on human health, and it will be in the area of food safety where integration of animal and human health will become most evident. Closer integration between veterinary and medical agencies provides ideal circumstances for ensuring effective liaison in the event of having to deal with the eventuality of an incursion by Rift Valley fever virus or indeed any hitherto unknown cause of haemorrhagic disease. The UK outbreak of foot and mouth disease in 2001 raised considerable issues of protecting the public, even though this virus is not known to cause human disease. Here the problem was the large scale burial of animal carcasses requiring the implementation of health protection measures that were complex and required co-ordination between government agencies at the highest level.

Urbanisation is now seen as one of the major contributory factors to disease emergence and evolution. The movement of peoples into cities has accelerated dramatically over the last 50 years, with present estimates of 75% of people in developed nations now dwelling in cities. Even in less economically developed countries this figure now exceeds 40%.[2] This is seen most dramatically in China where migration to the major cities continues unabated. As a marker of urbanisation, in 1975 there were just five cities where the number of inhabitants exceeded 10 million. Just 25 years later there are now 19 of these "megacities", 11 of them in Asia (United Nations Population Fund Report, 2001).

---

[1] Further details of the WHO Outbreak Alert and Response Network can be found at http://www.who.int/emc/index.html.

[2] United Nations Population Division survey.

As the majority of viral haemorrhagic fevers are zoonoses, it could be argued that increased dwelling in cities and towns would lessen the chance of exposure to existing or newly emerging zoonoses but this ignores the capacity for pathogens to evolve along with changing behaviour of hosts and reservoirs. Dengue is a prime example of a haemorrhagic fever that is no longer constrained by the dynamics of natural animal reservoirs. Childhood diseases, for example measles, have long been considered by some as originating in peridomestic animals but evolved independent of animal hosts once humans collectivised into townships. There are no obvious hurdles to prevent presently recognised viral haemorrhagic fevers—or indeed any other group of zoonoses—from crossing species barriers and becoming established in animals in closer proximity to town and city dwellers, to ultimately dispense with the need for a non-human reservoir. For this to happen would require a major change in transmissibility such that person-to-person transmission became the norm. The risk of this happening is greater for viruses with segmented genomes where a number of other viruses non-pathogenic for humans co-circulate. A warning this can be more than a theoretical consideration is provided by the emergence of Garissa virus in the Horn of Africa. Reassortment of gene segments has occurred between bunyamwera and a hitherto unidentified virus closely related to Cache Valley virus, leading to a widespread outbreak of disease among the local population and their livestock (Bowen et al. 2001). Host switching between rodent species is also occurring, particularly with respect to hantaviruses in North America, thus extending the range of these viruses and giving greater potential for changes in virulence.

Progressive urbanisation in turn accelerates change to the rural environment, both directly by economic forces driving the need for ever more intensive agriculture practices and indirectly by pollution influencing climatic change. Long-term weather patterns are a major factor in determining the habitat for small rodents and other reservoirs of infection, as shown so dramatically with the hantavirus outbreak of 1993 in the United States.

The rapid spread of HIV into populated and rural areas alike also has disturbed the symbiosis between infection and host species. Immunosuppression in a significant number of any given population must ultimately drive other pathogens to change in virulence and transmissibility. With the increase in urbanisation goes increasingly greater reliance on transport, with the propensity to disseminate both infected individuals, infected vectors and even infected host reservoirs.

Bioterrorism

Viral haemorrhagic fevers are amongst the group of pathogens assessed by the Centres of Disease Control as most likely posing a threat from bioterrorism (Table 1). The Working Group on Civilian Biodefense in the USA has identified a list of key features that characterise those pathogens in Category A that pose the greatest risk (Borio et al., 2002). Almost all of the viruses described in this monograph meet these criteria. The exception is dengue fever as it is not spread by small particle aerosols. The Working Group has also excluded Crimean-Congo haemorrhagic fever virus and hantaviruses on

Table 1

Categorisation of pathogens by the US Centres for Disease Control with potential as biological weapons (Rotz et al., 2002)

Category A	Category B	Category C
Variola major	*Coxiella burnetii*	Nipah virus
Bacillus anthracis	*Brucella* spp.	Hendra virus
Yersinia pestis	*Burkholderia mallei*	Hantaviruses
Clostridium botulinum	*Burkholderia pseudomallei*	
Francisella tularensis	Alphaviruses	
Filoviruses	*Rickettsia prowazekii*	
Arenaviruses	*Salmonella* spp., *E. coli* 0157:H7	
	Vibrio cholerae	
	Crytosporidium parvum	

the grounds that these agents are difficult to grow to sufficiently high titre in cell culture, making mass production unfeasible. Nevertheless, these agents have the potential to cause severe morbidity and mortality should the technical issues of large-scale production be resolved at some point in the future. Crimean-Congo haemorrhagic fever virus would then pose a particular threat as this virus spreads readily from person to person and has a high case fatality rate.

The use of viral haemorrhagic fevers as biological weapons is not a new concept. Both the former Soviet Union and the United States have indulged in the appropriate research programmes. The former Soviet Union is known to have had an active military driven programme from 1926 to 1992, during which time Marburg virus was developed as a weapon supported by research as to the potential offensive value of Ebola virus, those arenaviruses pathogenic for man, and yellow fever. The United States ran a similar programme from 1943 onwards although this was terminated in 1969 before the discovery of Marburg and Ebola viruses. Other countries declared as part of the Biological and Toxins Weapons Convention to have developed offensive biological weapons, including the United Kingdom, although the latter programme did not include any of the agents that cause haemorrhagic fever. Countries such as North Korea and Canada, along with the Soviet Union, contemplated the use of yellow fever as an offensive agent, despite the widespread use of a vaccine.

No doubt many other nations considered the use of biological weapons as a considerably cheaper alternative to nuclear or conventional weaponry. Large-scale facilities are not absolutely necessary and production can be easily disguised as part of legitimate medical and biological research programmes. Molecular biology now offers the option of developing pathogens with increased virulence or increased host range, or both. In the case of where vaccines are already available, e.g. yellow fever, specific mutations can be engineered to render the protective immunity induced by the presently available products as ineffective.

Biological weapons share along with nuclear and chemical weapons the epithet of weapons of mass destruction, a term so currently in vogue with politicians.

The Biological and Toxins Weapons Convention came into force in 1975, after which time all stockpiles were to be destroyed and fresh work on offensive biological and chemical weapons abandoned. Unfortunately, it became clear in the 1990s that a number of countries—including the former Soviet Union—had continued such programmes after having ratified the terms of the convention. The first sign of this was the sudden announcement by the Soviet President Yeltsin in 1992 that an anthrax outbreak which occurred in 1979 in Sverdlovsk was the result of accidental release of organisms being developed as part of a continuing programme of offensive biological research in the Soviet Union.

The importance of diagnostics

The United States has embarked upon a policy of "Syndromic Surveillance" whereupon data concerning trends in symptoms are monitored through sifting medical records of disease in the general population. Although this may indicate the possible ebb and flow of disease patterns through the seasons, it is a poor substitute for an enhanced and strengthened diagnostic capability for specific disease agents. Here the needs of the developed world contrast sharply with those of the poorer nations that history has shown as bearing the brunt of outbreaks. Rare incursions of infectious disease into the industrialised world can be dealt with by calling upon the resources and skills of national public health structures that can readily adapt existing platform technologies to the need of the moment.

Ideally a diagnosis is made by identifying the causative agent employing a method that does not start with any perceived notions as to the nature or the type of agent being sought. Electron microscopy is ideal for this purpose, especially for filoviruses and arenaviruses with a distinctive and unique morphology. It is rapid and, subject to the availability of appropriate antisera, adaptable for confirming the identity of an agent. An answer can be had in a matter of hours. The drawbacks are considerable, however: the equipment is expensive, cumbersome and a considerable supporting infrastructure is required for the preparation of samples. It suffers from artefacts and a lack of sensitivity and a skilled operator is an absolute requirement. Virus particles are seen in clinical specimens only if present at a high concentration. Notwithstanding these difficulties, electron microscopy still has an important role to play in diagnosing viral haemorrhagic fevers and other viral pathogens. Unfortunately, training in electron microscopy has become unfashionable and the expense of providing such facilities is constantly questioned.

Probe-specific assays for detecting virus genomes rely on nucleic acid extraction and amplification of duplexes initiated by addition of specific primers. As viral haemorrhagic fevers are RNA viruses, an initial reverse transcription step is required. No matter how able the investigator or efficient the protocol, direct detection of virus by PCR or hybridisation rarely detects the agent in more than 50–70% of acute phase samples. One advantage, however, is that extraction procedures are likely to inactivate any virus that may be present in the sample, although it must be stressed that such assays must be carried out within the confines of the appropriate biosafety laboratory.

Difficulties arise when primers give rise to false positive reactions as a result of self-priming. These non-specific reactions can be avoided by judicious selection of primer sequences and by confirming the size of the DNA product by gel electrophoresis. Increasing numbers of partial and complete gene sequences deposited in databanks mean that consensus sequences can now be identified with a greater level of confidence, thus increasing the chance of detecting a new agent with a well-characterised family of viruses. Sequences within the gene coding for the RNA polymerase are often the region of choice, together with genes coding for other non-structural proteins. In recent times, considerable experience has been obtained with the detection of hepatitis C virus using this approach.

Direct genome detection by any number of PCR-based assay formats can quickly narrow the search and give vital clues as to the type of immediate public health response needed for control and treatment. Even in the developed world, however, standardising reagents and primer sets for PCR analysis are fraught with the problems of sensitivity and standardisation.

The diagnostics industry is currently dominated by a few large companies. The thrust of these companies has been driven by advances in technology combined with ever greater interest in the exploitation of major opportunities in human genetics. The screening of blood donations for agents of viral hepatitis and HIV has stimulated much of the drive for rapid detection combined with high sensitivity. Smaller companies with a medical diagnostics focus have found it difficult to attract new investors into what has become a largely static market where commercial growth is perceived as most likely by a shift away from traditional diagnosis of acute infectious disease to the diagnosis of chronic infections, especially of the elderly. These factors exacerbate further the difficulties in engaging the commercial diagnostics sector and re-enforce the need for developing robust tests for both the developed and the developing world. The public sector could benefit from acquiring the freedom to operate using platform technologies licensed from industry with specific restrictions on their use for emerging and rare diseases. In particular, those technologies that deliver diagnosis at the point of care where initial diagnosis is more important than the sensitivity afforded by more sophisticated and expensive assays.

The situation is very different in the developing world, especially in Africa. Here national capacity is low at best but is more often absent. Even when supplemented by the help of international agencies, the use of sophisticated molecular assays is out of the question. The need in these areas is for robust serological assays with long shelve life and minimal dependency on expensive equipment for obtaining a read out. Even ELISA can prove difficult to use as many African sera contain high levels of non-specific inhibitors. Tests such as reverse passive haemagglutination proved more robust for serological surveys of, e.g. hepatitis B as the reagents could be freeze-dried.

Prospects for better treatment

There are no antiviral compounds presently licensed for use against viral haemorrhagic fevers, although ribavirin, a nucleoside analogue, has been used in the treatment of the South American arenaviruses and HFRS. The major mechanism of action is the induction of error-prone replication leading to a cessation of RNA synthesis, but other indirect effects, e.g. on translation efficiency of viral mRNA, may contribute to an overall reduction in viral load. The difficulty in practice is that larger quantities need to be given than is indicated for the treatment of respiratory infections, for which this drug is approved. However, intravenous ribavirin is in very short supply. Ribavirin also induces a haemolytic anaemia in a dose-dependent manner which in turn can lead to cardiac and pulmonary complications, thereby restricting its potential use still further. Animal studies also have shown a teratogenic effect in several species, thus ribavirin is not advised for use in pregnant women. There are improved derivatives of ribavirin under development that may overcome some of these issues of dosage and unwanted side effects. With the exception of the study by Huggins et al. (1991), there have not been adequate controlled trials, and in any event ribavirin is not effective against filoviruses. Although not effective against yellow fever and dengue, it has been used for the treatment of chronic hepatitis C in combination with α-interferon, hepatitis C virus also being a member of the Flaviviridae family. Unfortunately, ribavirin exacerbates the interferon-induced fatigue, and may be accompanied by other side effects, such as a rash or irritating cough. Long acting interferons have been produced with the chronic hepatitis C market very much in mind. These are recombinant interferon preparations linked to polyethylene glycopolymers (PEG), giving a marked long-term improvement in clinical outcome (Manns et al., 2001). These products may be worth considering for the treatment of isolated cases of viral haemorrhagic disease in combination with ribavirin, but the considerable expense of this therapy places this treatment well beyond the means of those in developing countries.

It is thus clear that a new generation of compounds is urgently needed, perhaps exploiting other inhibitory pathways, such as inhibiting viral-specific proteases or RNA polymerase. In this context, viral haemorrhagic research will undoubtedly benefit from the intensive efforts currently in finding new drugs against HIV and hepatitis C virus (HCV). There are several new compounds that block the nucleotide-binding catalytic domain of the HCV polymerase NS5B. These non-nucleotide inhibitors (NNIs) show considerable promise and are the subject of early clinical trials. The similarity between HCV RNA ploymerase structure and at least the NS5B of other flaviviruses, may offer scope for new compounds against viral haemorrhagic fevers, the majority of the development costs having been borne by programmes targeting other diseases where the market can adsorb these expenses in the product price. Equally promising is a potent competitive inhibitor of NS3–NS4A complex of HCV, but again the potential for treating other RNA virus infections will be dependent upon the outcome of clinical trials in patients with chronic hepatitis C. An entirely different approach is the blocking of virus attachment to cellular receptors. One way of achieving this has been proposed by Barrientos et al. (2003) who showed that cyanovirin-B, a derivative from the cyanobacterium *Nostoc ellipsosporium*, binds with high affinity to Ebola glycoproteins rich in mannose oligosaccharides. Furthermore, such binding reduced significantly in a mice model both the onset of illness and the mean time of death.

There is much excitement as to the therapeutic potential of small interfering RNA (siRNA) molecules since it was discovered that gene silencing in plants also occurred in mammalian cells. These short, ~ 22 bp double-stranded RNA structures interact with the host argonaute proteins; the double-stranded structure then unwinds to reveal a single-stranded RNA molecule specific for the target sequence, which is subsequently degraded (Hannon, 2002). Hepatitis C virus, a member of the Flaviviridae family, is sensitive to RNA interference (Randall et al., 2003) so there is every reason to expect that a similar approach could be found for designing siRNAs with activity against other flaviviruses and RNA viruses in general. However, even if such siRNA molecules are shown to be effective against viruses such as Lassa and Ebola, the problem will be one of delivery. RNAs are inherently unstable in cells and in the circulation. There would also be concerns regarding escape mutations. Notwithstanding these issues, circumstances may well develop over the next decade whereby drug delivery systems are successfully modified for the delivery of RNA, thus overcoming the present difficulties of targeting nucleic acid therapies to infected tissues.

The use of immunoglobulin for post-exposure prophylaxis was pioneered by the late Dr Julio Maiztegui and his colleagues in the 1970s (Enria et al., 1984a). Although specific for Junin infections, this work broke new ground, showing the use of immune plasma to have considerable potential for treatment provided high titres of virus neutralising antibodies were present. For viruses such as Junin and others where there is well-documented evidence of neutralising antibodies, there are grounds for considering the development of therapeutic antibodies. In addition to humanising murine antibodies, there are now a myriad of approaches towards antibody engineering. For example, cytokines can be linked to antibody fragments, bispecific antibodies can be designed that recognise two different epitopes, or antibodies integrated into liposome delivery vehicles that contain other therapeutic agents (Presta, 2003).

For pursuing any or all of the above approaches to maximum benefit, there needs to be a perception on the part of funding agencies that the agents of haemorrhagic disease constitute a funding priority. It is unlikely in the present economic climate that the pharmaceutical industry will pursue any novel approach when the costs of development are so high and the potential returns so limited, with the possible exception of new agents for treating dengue. Ultimately progress will only be made by harnessing platform technologies for use in the public sector against clearly defined target diseases and potential markets.

Vaccine development

Vaccination is often suggested as a priority for controlling viral haemorrhagic fevers. The ultimate goal for any immunisation strategy is to interrupt disease transmission. For this to happen the level of vaccine coverage among susceptible members of the population must be high and it must be sustained over many years. It is difficult to see how such a situation can ever be achieved for the viral haemorrhagic fevers other than perhaps yellow fever—and once a polyvalent vaccine is available—dengue.

All is not gloom, however, as there have been some notable successes in the control of viral haemorrhagic fevers. Yellow fever vaccines have been spectacularly successful in eliminating this disease from many areas of the world. A safe and highly effective vaccine has been available since 1937 and until 30 years ago its use combined with vector control kept this disease firmly at bay. Yet every year there are at least 200,000 cases and about 30,000 deaths, many of them children. Of the 37 countries at high risk of yellow fever, only 26 have included the vaccine as part of the routine immunisation of infants. The problem is particularly severe in Africa where there is a lack of awareness as to the burden of disease, coupled with a lack of capacity to run an effective immunisation programme. The stocks of 17D vaccine seed lots are low and the technology used to produce master lots is heavily dependent upon the use of embryonated eggs. Attempts to adapt 17D virus to cell culture have been unsuccessful: the yield is simply too low for producing a vaccine product on the sufficiently large scale required and the cost per dose would be considerable. In 2000 an outbreak in Guinea in West Africa involving over 800 cases subsequently led to an international effort directed towards rapid control by immunisation, and in the process seriously depleted the global stocks of 17D vaccine.

Increasing urbanisation, overcrowding and poverty plus the abandoning of mosquito control programmes mean there is now a real fear of explosive outbreaks in large conurbations. In 1988, the World Health Organisation recommended that yellow fever vaccine is added to the existing list of childhood vaccines for the 20 million children borne each year in Africa. The challenge of immunising children in the developing world against the six most common childhood diseases of early life is considerable. The World Health Organisation has a target of 90% of the world's children should have access to vaccines financed by their own governments. A study in 1993 showed that routine vaccination could be seven times as effective in reducing the number of cases as hastily organised mass immunisation programmes organised in the face of an epidemic. Although initial enthusiasm saw a good start to the introduction of yellow fever vaccine, initial encouragement of coverage rates as 87% (in The Gambia) and 51% (in Burkino Faso) has now slumped to depressingly low levels. This is against the backdrop of an estimated 200,000 cases per year in sub-Saharan Africa. Unfortunately the poorest nations continue to depend upon international donors for providing access to these vaccines.

The problems of implementing any vaccination programme are twofold. First, there is the issue of funding. The second is the matter of the low perception of vaccines as opposed to treatment once an infection has taken hold. This gross distortion on curing the sick at great cost rather than preventing the infection in the first place with vaccines that cost little precludes the development of more esoteric vaccines on diseases such as Ebola and Lassa fever.

Who would be vaccinated, and against what disease? African countries stand much to gain from the introduction of vaccines against Ebola and Lassa fever. Were such vaccines to be developed the question is: who would pay for their use in some of the poorest nations of the world where total healthcare expenditure for every man, woman and child is often less than $6 per year? In 2001 the World Health Organisation sponsored a Commission on Macroeconomics and Health that declared a nation must spend at least $30 per year per capita to maintain even the very basic level of health care for its population. The odds are stacked against such countries reaching a basic level of infrastructure able to cope with immunisation programmes targeting the common diseases of childhood, let alone developing the capacity for controlling unexpected outbreaks of haemorrhagic fevers.

There is every indication that vaccines against Ebola may eventually be developed if the recent excitement using a single dose of recombinant adenovirus expressing the glycoprotein of Ebola withstands the test of further animal challenge testing and safety testing in humans. The major problems are defining the correlates of protection in humans and circumventing the need for full-scale efficacy studies. With respect to the latter, there are precedents: hepatitis A vaccines, for example, were licensed before large-scale efficacy data became available. It is almost inconceivable that anything other than a recombinant (subunit) protein or a whole particle, inactivated vaccine will be accepted for human use. Much the same applies to viruses such as Lassa fever and the bunyaviruses. What is needed is a concerted international effort that engages both academia and the private sector: the World Health Organisation is well placed in this respect and indeed has targeted dengue vaccines as among its priorities for preventing tropical diseases.

Newer technologies including DNA immunisation offer considerable scope for use in the developing world as potential vaccines based on the use of DNA expressing specific gene products are cheaply produced and easily stored for long periods. The drawback is that human trials employing DNA expressing, e.g. influenza proteins have proved considerably less immunogenic in humans compared to mice. The development of appropriate delivery vehicles may provide the answer to enhancing the immunogenic potential of such immunogens.

Conclusion

Viral haemorrhagic fevers remain as important to public health as when first described in the mid-20th century. An even greater number of these viruses are likely to emerge in the years to come with at best the endemic areas of existing agents of viral haemorrhagic fever confined to existing geographical areas and ecosystems. The only certainty is that more of these agents will be discovered as mankind continues to alter the environment and with it the balance between humans and those species with which we share the planet. Although we know in ever increasing detail the molecular events accompanying their replication—and even the detail of certain protein structures at the Ångstrom level—we have made little progress with understanding just how these agents can cause devastating human disease. Where viruses such as Ebola and Marburg come from remains one of the great mysteries of microbiology. Until more is known as to their epidemiology, finding appropriate means of prevention and developing a strategy for effective control will remain as elusive as ever. Just how mankind's relentless pursuit of altering and abusing the environment triggers outbreaks of these viruses will continue to challenge both infectious disease specialists and public health officials alike for many decades to come.

Those among our societies with the remit of pursuing these challenges need to recognise the imperative of convincing politicians at all levels that such efforts require adequate resources and sufficient numbers of trained personnel. Above all, the argument needs to be enumerated in terms of the cost benefit to communities and governments convinced that complacency threatens the very fabric of society. Equally the scientific community has to make more effort to ensure the public is better informed regarding infectious diseases and, where appropriate, take steps to allay fears regarding the use of vaccines. We can only hope that sufficient resources are forthcoming to ensure we react swiftly, thus minimising the risk of outbreaks disseminating and quickly overwhelming public health infrastructures in the developing and developed world alike.

Appendix 1: Useful sources of information on the Worldwide Web

The Internet now provides a rich source of up-to-date information on agents causing viral haemorrhagic disease. The list below, whilst not comprehensive, will give the reader access to a variety of sources and include links directing the enquirer to other websites with specific details.

International Committee for the Taxonomy of Viruses Database (ICTVdB) (http://www.ncbi.nlm.nih.gov/ICTVdb/)

For the latest descriptions of all the viruses described in this book (general properties, specific features of the genera, and lists of GenBank accession numbers of sequences and representative genomes), see the online version of the 7th Report of the International Committee for the Taxonomy of Viruses (ICTV). An invaluable source of basic information, particularly useful for learning of accepted data regarding the molecular properties of virus.

World Health Organisation (http://www.who.int)

This site contains detailed information regarding outbreaks and surveillance. Useful also for obtaining summary reports of consultative meetings sponsored by WHO.

United States Centres for Disease Control (http://www.cdc.gov/ncidod/)

A very comprehensive site providing much basic information supplemented by a variety of teaching materials that can be downloaded and used for training. Also useful in providing guidance notes for the safe handling of pathogens and the care of patients suspected of having a viral haemorrhagic fever.

United States National Library of Medicine (http://www.nlm.nih.gov)

Much more than a library, this site gives access to detailed information concerning the NCBI database of genome and protein sequences. The primary source of bibliographic material for this book.

ProMED-mail (http://www.promedmail.org)

This site is maintained by the International Society for Infectious Diseases. Regular email alerts are available. The first site experts in the filed of emerging diseases visit for up-to-date information on outbreaks around the world. Known to have information posted before the same data became available locally!

Appendix 2: Further reading

Ebola: A Documentary Novel of its First Explosion by William T. Close, Ivy Books, New York, 1995, ISBN 0-8041-1432-3.

Although written as a novel, this book is based on the facts surrounding the first reported cases of Ebola in Zaire. Dr William Close was a physician for 16 years in Zaire and involved at close quarters with the handling of the 1976 Yambuku outbreak. He worked for many years in Zambia, and thus this book gives an accurate rendering of the landscape and communities most affected by Ebola during the early days, and how the first teams came to terms with the difficulties in controlling a disease hitherto unrecognised by western medicine.

The History of Yellow Fever: An Essay on the Birth of Tropical Medicine by François Delaporte, 1991, The MIT Press, Cambridge, 0-262-04112-X.

The discovery that yellow fever was transmitted by the bite of a mosquito and the circumstances surrounding this discovery by Walter Reed and his colleagues have long fascinated historians. This book examines the background to its discovery and likely influences from other 19th century specialists in tropical diseases.

Fever! The Hunt for a New Killer Virus by John G. Fuller, Hart-Davis, MacGibbon, London, 1974, ISBN 0-246-10840-1.

This account of how Lassa fever emerged in the late 1960s is a mix of graphic detail of the early cases written with the human dimension very much in mind. Unusual for a book written for the lay reader, it contains a useful bibliography of the early scientific and medical literature. Essential reading for those interested in the early days of haemorrhagic fever research.

Yellow Fever and the South by Margaret Humphreys, The Johns Hopkins University press, Baltimore, 1999, ISBN 0-8018-6196-9.

A detailed historiographical account of how yellow fever influenced trade and settlement in the southern states during the 19th century.

The Virus Hunters: Dispatches from the Front Line by Joseph B. McCormick and Susan Fisher-Hoch, Bloomsbury, London, 1996, ISBN 0-7475-3030-0.

Probably two of the most experienced clinicians in the diagnosis and treatment of haemorrhagic disease, this account is unusual in that each author has written alternative chapters.

Viruses, Plagues and History by Michael B.A. Oldstone, Oxford University Press, New York, 1998, ISBN 0-19-511723-9.

Although not confined to viral haemorrhagic fevers, this book gives a general introduction to viruses and how throughout the last two centuries societies have had to come to terms with the ravages of infectious diseases. The chapter on yellow fever in the

Americas is particularly useful as background to modern day concerns as to the risk this virus continues to pose. Other chapters include descriptions of the early Lassa fever outbreaks and the more recent emergence of hantavirus infections in the United States.

Virus Hunter: Thirty years of Battling Hot Viruses Around the World by C.J. Peters and Mark Olshaker, Anchor Books, New York, 1997, ISBN 0-385-48557-3.

Essentially an autobiography, C.J. Peters more than any other specialist in viral haemorrhagic fevers has attempted to set his scientific world in the context of a personal voyage through life with all its attendant joys and disappointments.

The Hot Zone by Richard Preston, Random House, New York, 1994, ISBN 0-679-43094-6.

More than any other book of its genre, Preston's account of how the Reston outbreak of Ebola was dealt with in one of Washington's suburbs brought home to the public just how vulnerable even the most economically-advanced societies are to the threat of serious infectious disease. Events at Reston served to illustrate vividly how the scientists also must learn to deal with the political consequences of containment and quarantine. This book was the stimulus for Hollywood's box office success "Outbreak", starring Dustin Hoffman.

Scientific and medical books

Exotic Viral Diseases: A Global Guide by Stephen Berger, Charles H. Calisher and Jay Keystone, BC Decker, Montreal, 2003, ISBN 1-55009-205-7.

This truly pocket-sized guide is aimed for the clinician and others who need to keep a quick reference guide within easy reach. The descriptions are succinct but informative, encompassing the epidemiology, clinical signs and treatment options for all of the viral haemorrhagic fevers known to date. An added bonus is that it includes a CD-ROM with all of the information in PDF format.

Field's Virology (4th edn.) eds. Knipe, D.M. and Howley, P.M., Lippincott Williams & Wilkins, Philadelphia, 2001, IBSN 0-7817-1832-5.

Long regarded as the essential textbook on the molecular properties of viruses and the pathogenesis of virus diseases, this reference work contains extensive descriptions and bibliographies of all the viruses described in this book. There are also general introductory chapters reviewing the general properties and replication for those readers requiring a rapid introduction to virology.

Principles and Practice of Clinical Virology (5th edn.) eds. Zuckerman, A.J., Banatvala, J.E., Pattison, J.R., Schoub, B., and Griffiths, P., 2004, John Wiley & Sons Ltd, Chichester, ISBN 0-70-84338-1.

Recently revised, this remains an excellent introduction to the principles of diagnostic virology with overview chapters on all of the viruses described in this book. Particularly useful for those working in a hospital setting.

Zoonoses, ed. Palmer, S.R., Soulsby, L. and Simpson, D.I.H. Oxford University Press, 1998, ISBN 0-19-262380-X.

Useful review articles that include reviews on non-viral causes of disease that could be confused with viral haemorrhagic fevers in the early stages.

Appendix 3: Microbiological containment—a brief overview

The purpose of microbiological containment laboratories is to prevent and control the exposure of laboratory workers, other personnel and the external environment from biologically hazardous agents. The levels of containment relate directly to the perceived risk of human infection, the availability of prophylaxis and transmissibility. Additional considerations include the quantity of pathogen being handled, whether laboratory animals are involved in the procedure, and to what extent prior knowledge of the material can reasonably expect the presence of infectious hazard. This last consideration is particularly important when handling routine clinical samples where a range of microbiological causes are being investigated.

The handling of hazardous pathogens is subject to strict government regulations and legislation in the vast majority of countries in which such laboratories operate. The following are guidelines and serve to illustrate general principles. All those working with, and those intending to work with, any of the pathogens described in this book must refer to local authorities for guidance and be aware of national and local procedures prescribed by law. Where such guidance does not exist workers should seek guidance from international authorities such as the World Health Organisation, Switzerland or Centers for Disease Control, USA.

Containment operates in two ways. First, by the provision of suitable laboratories and safety equipment, e.g. microbiological containment safety cabinets. Second, by the adoption of good microbiological practices and techniques. Although immunisation should always be practised if vaccines are available, the use of preventative prophylaxis should never be relied upon as a primary means of protecting laboratory workers and certainly never as a substitute for those procedures commensurate with good microbiological practice.

Facilities are accorded one of four grades according to the level of containment offered, with 1 being the lowest and 4 the highest in terms of containment. These levels are briefly summarised in Table A3.1. It should be noted that there is some variation in the exact definition of these levels between different regulatory authorities. Those levels most relevant to the handling of viral haemorrhagic fevers are levels 3 and 4. The following provides a brief description of level 3 laboratories, the most commonly used facility for the handling of specimens, particularly those suspected of harbouring an unknown or dangerous pathogen. The design and operation of a level 4 facility, required for the specialist handling of many viruses described in this book, owes as much to engineering as it does to microbiology. As such the specialist features of a level 4 laboratory are only attained by few centres in the world and therefore are not described in detail.

Table A3.1

Categorisation of microbiological containment laboratories

Category[a]	Features	Usage
Level 1	General laboratory area: readily decontaminated surfaces and floors. Hand washing facilities available. Autoclave nearby	Agents not known to cause disease in healthy adults. Minimum potential hazard to personnel and the environment
Level 2	Laboratory area with restricted access: good microbiological practice in operation. Not used for other purposes. Sealed flooring and benches. Facilities for decontamination. Level suitable for routine diagnostic evaluation of clinical samples. Use of class II cabinets for work potentially generating aerosols or splashes	Pathogens of moderate potential human hazard. Immunisation and/or antibiotics available
Level 3	Restricted access to authorised users. Negative pressure airflow. Use of safety microbiological cabinets to contain aerosols. Dedicated equipment for analysis. Separate decontamination protocols	Pathogens that may cause serious or potentially fatal disease as a result of aerosol exposure
Level 4	All the features of a level 3 laboratory but with enhanced levels of decontamination and security. Showering of personnel on exit. Treatment of effluent. Workers in some facilities wear suits with independent air supply ("space suits")	Pathogens that may cause potentially fatal disease in healthy adults. No known therapy or vaccine available

[a]Biological Safety Level (BSL; United States) or Containment Level (CL; United Kingdom).

Design and layout

Rooms dedicated to level 3 activities should ideally be placed well away from areas visited by the general public and under negative pressure. Approximately 6–12 air changes per hour are required. An anteroom serves as an air lock where dedicated protective clothing can be stored. Work in the containment laboratory should be restricted to registered personnel only and entry allowed only by use of a swipe card or entry code. All areas of the laboratory should be clearly visible from service corridors and/or the entry point. Layout of equipment is important, especially the location of microbiological safety cabinets. At level 3, these represent the major source of airflow in the laboratory and thus must be sited so that movement across a cabinet threshold is minimised. A suitable vent in the door is required to ensure negative air pressure is maintained.

The flooring should be impermeable and sealed on a regular basis. Edges should be lipped and sealed at all skirting boards, allowing no opportunity for liquids to penetrate. Work surfaces should be resistant to acid, alkali, solvents and disinfectants. Ideally these should be made of solid plastic laminate material ("Trespar" or similar) and again edges sealed to prevent seepage of liquids into joints. Although varnished wood can meet the minimum specifications, its use is to be avoided whenever possible as wooden work surfaces quickly deteriorate. Sinks are best made of epoxy resin or polypropylene as stainless steel is susceptible to corrosion by disinfectants. Porcelain sinks should never be used.

A wash hand basin close to the exit door is a must and never used for any purpose other than for hand washing. The use of a good bactericidal hand soap is recommended preferably from a wall-mounted dispenser. Hands should always be dried on disposable towels.

Decontamination of material represents one of the major challenges in the use of containment laboratories. Electrical autoclaves within the containment laboratory are often used. Level 4 laboratories need a much more extensive waste treatment system, often provided by use of double-ended autoclaves. At level 4, all effluent also needs to be treated before it can be discharged into the local sewerage system.

Air handling

The laboratory must be maintained at a negative air pressure with respect to the external environment. This aspect is critical to level 3 and level 4 laboratories. If within a building with ducted ventilation, it is important that some mechanical system is present to prevent reverse airflows. The air handling system should be capable of isolation from the outside so that the laboratory can be fumigated. External instruments monitoring airflow are also desirable. The air temperature must be comfortable and the design should take account of heat generated by equipment located inside the laboratory. In tropical areas, this may require the use of a separate air conditioning unit that circulates cooled air back into the room. Air extracted from the laboratory needs to pass through a high efficiency particulate filter (HEPA) before being vented into the external atmosphere.

Safety cabinets

A microbiological safety cabinet is a ventilated enclosure designed primarily to protect the operator and the environment from aerosols generated when handling human pathogens. The effectiveness of microbiological safety cabinets depends critically on good design, correct use and regular maintenance. Proper installation and testing is vital. All need venting through one or more HEPA filters. There are several categories of microbiological safety cabinet. These are summarised in Table A3.2.

The effectiveness of safety cabinets can be seriously compromised by cluttering the work surface with plasticware and small items of equipment. Only what is needed for the

Table A3.2

Classification of microbiological safety cabinets

Category	Basic features
Class I	Escape of airborne particles contained by the flow of air through an open front aperture, normally the length of the cabinet. Not suited to protecting the material from adventitious contamination or for the handling of category 4 pathogens
Class II	Constructed with an open aperture but offers additional protection for the material being handled from adventitious contamination. Air drawn through the front aperture is filtered prior to flow over the work surface. Not suited for work with category 4 pathogens
Class III	The work area is completely enclosed, accessible only by use of integral rubber gloves attached to the front ports. Air entering and venting the cabinet is filtered through one or more HEPA filters. Usually confined to work with category 4 pathogens

procedure in hand should be placed within the cabinet and the whole cabinet cleared after a working session. The use of Bunsen burners within cabinets should be discouraged as their use disrupts severely the laminar flow of air across the work surface. In practice, many laboratories leave cabinets running for a set period of time between sessions.

Apart from meeting safety standards, it is worth thinking carefully about operator comfort. The work surface within the cabinet needs to be well lit and the front edge facing the operator needs to accommodate the wrists without undue discomfort. Some workers find cabinets with large filter units facing out over the operator's head a distraction. The laboratory stool needs to be the best available and consideration given to side benches for temporary storage of equipment whilst the cabinet is in use. In practice, the use of two or more cabinets abutting each other is to be avoided as this design quickly leads to clutter with the attendant risk of cross-contamination.

Protective clothing

Dedicated laboratory coats are required. These should not be used in other laboratories and never worn in areas visited by the general public. Coats should be closed at the side of the body and fastened securely around the neck. Elasticated wrists ensure normal clothing does not come into contact with work surfaces. Laboratory coats of a different colour to those used in other laboratories are often used. Good quality disposable gloves are a must, and should be available in a range of sizes. Other protective clothing may be necessary according to the risk assessment, such as disposable gowns, aprons, disposable overshoes and masks. Masks should meet the requirements of the N-95 standard. Goggles or a visor for eye protection is essential. It is advisable to remove items of jewellery and other personal items. Level 4 laboratories also require a complete change of clothing and a shower on exit.

Further reading

Advisory Committee on Dangerous Pathogens. The Management, Design and Operation of Microbiological Containment Laboratories. London: Her Majesty's Stationery Office; 2001; ISBN 0-7176-2034-4.

http://www.hse.gov.uk/pubns/misc208.pdf

Richmond JY, McKinney RW. Biosafety in Microbiological and Biomedical Laboratories. 4th ed. Washington, DC: US Government Printing Office; 1999.

http://www.cdc.gov/od/ohs/biosfty

World Health Organisation. Laboratory Biosafety Manual. 2nd ed. Geneva 1993; ISBN 9-241-54450-3.

http://www.who.int/csr/resources/publications/biosafety

References

Albarino CG, Posik DM, Ghiringhelli PD, Lozano ME, Romanowski V. Arenavirus phylogeny: a new insight. Virus Genes 1998; 16(1): 39–46.

Alvarez CP, Lasala F, Carrillo J, Muniz O, Corbi AL, Delgado R. C-type lectins DC-SIGN and L-SIGN mediate cellular entry by Ebola virus in cis and in trans. J Virol 2002; 76(13): 6841–6844.

Ambrosio AM, Feuillade MR, Gamboa GS, Maiztegui JI. Prevalence of lymphocytic choriomeningitis virus infection in a human population of Argentina. Am J Trop Med Hyg 1994; 50(3): 381–386.

An J, Kimura-Kuroda J, Hirabayashi Y, Yasui K. Development of a novel mouse model for dengue virus infection. Virology 1999; 263(1): 70–77.

Anderson GW Jr, Slone TW Jr, Peters CJ. Pathogenesis of Rift Valley fever virus (RVFV) in inbred rats. Microb Pathog 1987; 2(4): 283–293.

Anderson ED, Thomas L, Hayflick JS, Thomas G. Inhibition of HIV-1 gp160-dependent membrane fusion by a furin-directed alpha 1-antitrypsin variant. J Biol Chem 1993; 268(33): 24887–24891.

Andrei G, De Clercq E. Molecular approaches for the treatment of hemorrhagic fever virus infections. Antivir Res 1993; 22(1): 45–75.

Barnard BJ. Rift Valley fever vaccine—antibody and immune response in cattle to a live and an inactivated vaccine. J S Afr Vet Assoc 1979; 50(3): 155–157.

Barnard BJ, Botha MJ. An inactivated rift valley fever vaccine. J S Afr Vet Assoc 1977; 48(1): 45–48.

Barrett AD. Yellow fever vaccines. Biologicals 1997; 25(1): 17–25.

Barrientos LG, O'Keefe BR, Bray M, Sanchez A, Gronenborn AM, Boyd MR. Cyanovirin-N binds to the viral surface glycoprotein, GP1,2 and inhibits infectivity of Ebola virus. Antivir Res 2003; 58(1): 47–56.

Baskerville A, Fisher-Hoch SP, Neilds GH, Dowsett AB. Ultrastructure pathology of experimental Ebola haemorrhagic fever virus infection. J Pathol 1985; 147: 199–209.

Bausch DG, Rollin PE, Demby AH, Coulibaly M, Kanu J, Conteh AS, Wagoner KD, McMullan LK, Bowen MD, Peters CJ, Ksiazek TG. Diagnosis and clinical virology of Lassa fever as evaluated by enzyme-linked immunosorbent assay, indirect fluorescent-antibody test, and virus isolation. J Clin Microbiol 2000; 38(7): 2670–2677.

Bavari S, Bosio CM, Wiegand E, Ruthel G, Will AB, Geisbert TW, Hevey M, Schmaljohn C, Schmaljohn A, Aman MJ. Lipid raft microdomains: a gateway for compartmentalized trafficking of Ebola and Marburg viruses. J Exp Med 2002; 195(5): 593–602.

Blaney JE Jr, Johnson DH, Firestone CY, Hanson CT, Murphy BR, Whitehead SS. Chemical mutagenesis of dengue virus type 4 yields mutant viruses which are temperature sensitive in vero cells or human liver cells and attenuated in mice. J Virol 2001; 75(20): 9731–9740.

Bockstahler LE, Carney PG, Bushar G, Sagripanti JL. Detection of Junin virus by the polymerase chain reaction. J Virol Methods 1992; 39(1–2): 231–235.

Borden KL, Campbell Dwyer EJ, Salvato MS. An arenavirus RING (zinc-binding) protein binds the oncoprotein promyelocyte leukemia protein (PML) and relocates PML nuclear bodies to the cytoplasm. J Virol 1998; 72(1): 758–766.

Borio L, Inglesby T, Peters CJ, Schmaljohn AL, Hughes JM, Jahrling PB, Ksiazek T, Johnson KM, Meyerhoff A, O'Toole T, Ascher MS, Bartlett J, Breman JG, Eitzen EM Jr, Hamburg M, Hauer J, Henderson DA, Johnson RT, Kwik G, Layton M, Lillibridge S, Nabel GJ, Osterholm MT, Perl TM, Russell P, Tonat K. Hemorrhagic fever viruses as biological weapons: medical and public health management. J Am Med Assoc 2002; 287(18): 2391–2405.

Bowen MD, Peters CJ, Mills JN, Nichol ST. Oliveros virus: a novel arenavirus from Argentina. Virology 1996; 217(1): 362–366.

Bowen MD, Peters CJ, Nichol ST. Phylogenetic analysis of the Arenaviridae: patterns of virus evolution and evidence for cospeciation between arenaviruses and their rodent hosts. Mol Phylogenet Evol 1997; 8(3): 301–316.

Bowen MD, Rollin PE, Ksiazek TG, Hustad HL, Bausch DG, Demby AH, Bajani MD, Peters CJ, Nichol ST. Genetic diversity among Lassa virus strains. J Virol 2000; 74(15): 6992–7004.

Bowen MD, Trappier SG, Sanchez AJ, Meyer RF, Goldsmith CS, Zaki SR, Dunster LM, Peters CJ, Ksiazek TG, Nichol ST. A re assortant bunyavirus isolated from acute hemorrhagic fever cases in Kenya and Somalia. Virology 2001; 291(2): 185–190.

Bray M, Lai CJ. Construction of intertypic chimeric dengue viruses by substitution of structural protein genes. Proc Natl Acad Sci USA 1991; 88(22): 10342–10346.

Bridson E. The English 'sweate' (Sudor Anglicus) and Hantavirus pulmonary syndrome. Br J Biomed Sci 2001; 58(1): 1–6.

Brinkworth RI, Fairlie DP, Leung D, Young PR. Homology model of the dengue 2 virus NS3 protease: putative interactions with both substrate and NS2B cofactor. J Gen Virol 1999; 80(Pt 5): 1167–1177.

Brus SK, Golovljova I, Plyusnin A, Lundkvist A. Diagnostic potential of puumala virus nucleocapsid protein expressed in *Drosophila melanogaster* cells. J Clin Microbiol 2000; 38(6): 2324–2329.

Buchmeier MJ, Lewicki HA, Tomori O, Oldstone MB. Monoclonal antibodies to lymphocytic choriomeningitis and pichinde viruses: generation, characterization, and cross-reactivity with other arenaviruses. Virology 1981; 113(1): 73–85.

Burt FJ, Swanepoel R, Shieh WJ, Smith JF, Leman PA, Greer PW, Coffield LM, Rollin PE, Ksiazek TG, Peters CJ, Zaki SR. Immunohistochemical and in situ localization of Crimean-Congo hemorrhagic fever (CCHF) virus in human tissues and implications for CCHF pathogenesis. Arch Pathol Lab Med 1997; 121(8): 839–846.

Camicas JL, Cornet JP, Gonzalez JP, Wilson ML, Adam F, Zeller HG. Crimean-Congo hemorrhagic fever in Senegal Latest data on the ecology of the CCHF virus. Bull Soc Pathol Exot 1994; 87(1): 11–16.

Cao W, Henry MD, Borrow P, Yamada H, Elder JH, Ravkov EV, Nichol ST, Compans RW, Campbell KP, Oldstone MB. Identification of alpha-dystroglycan as a receptor for lymphocytic choriomeningitis virus and Lassa fever virus. Science 1998; 282(5396): 2079–2081.

Caplen H, Peters CJ, Bishop DH. Mutagen-directed attenuation of Rift Valley fever virus as a method for vaccine development. J Gen Virol 1985; 66(Pt 10): 2271–2277.

Carey DE, Kemp GE, White HA, Pinneo L, Addy RF, Fom AL, Stroh G, Casals J, Henderson BE. Lassa fever. Epidemiological aspects of the 1970 epidemic, Jos, Nigeria. Trans R Soc Trop Med Hyg 1972; 66(3): 402–408.

Casals J. Arenaviruses. Yale J Biol Med 1975; 48(2): 115–140.

Chang GJ, Cropp BC, Kinney RM, Trent DW, Gubler DJ. Nucleotide sequence variation of the envelope protein gene identifies two distinct genotypes of yellow fever virus. J Virol 1995; 69(9): 5773–5780.

Chapman LE, Mertz GJ, Peters CJ, Jolson HM, Khan AS, Ksiazek TG, Koster FT, Baum KF, Rollin PE, Pavia AT, Holman RC, Christenson JC, Rubin PJ, Behrman RE, Bell LJ, Simpson GL, Sadek RF, Ribavirin Study Group. Intravenous ribavirin for hantavirus pulmonary syndrome: safety and tolerance during 1 year of open-label experience. Antivir Ther 1999; 4(4): 211–219.

Charrel RN, de Lamballerie X, Fulhorst CF. The Whitewater Arroyo virus: natural evidence for genetic recombination among Tacaribe serocomplex viruses (family Arenaviridae). Virology 2001; 283(2): 161–166.

Charrel RN, Zaki AM, Attoui H, Fakeeh M, Billoir F, Yousef AI, de Chesse R, De Micco P, Gould EA, de Lamballerie X. Complete coding sequence of the Alkhurma virus, a tick-borne flavivirus causing severe hemorrhagic fever in humans in Saudi Arabia. Biochem Biophys Res Commun 2001; 287(2): 455–461.

Chen Y, Maguire T, Hileman RE, Fromm JR, Esko JD, Linhardt RJ, Marks RM. Dengue virus infectivity depends on envelope protein binding to target cell heparan sulfate. Nat Med 1997; 3(8): 866–871.

Chen YC, Wang SY, King CC. Bacterial lipopolysaccharide inhibits dengue virus infection of primary human monocytes/macrophages by blockade of virus entry via a CD14-dependent mechanism. J Virol 1999; 73(4): 2650–2657.

Chiewsilp P, Scott RM, Bhamarapravati N. Histocompatibility antigens and dengue hemorrhagic fever. Am J Trop Med Hyg 1981; 30(5): 1100–1105.

Childs JE, Glass GE, Ksiazek TG, Rossi CA, Oro JG, LeDuc JW. Human–rodent contact and infection with lymphocytic choriomeningitis and Seoul viruses in an inner-city population. Am J Trop Med Hyg 1991; 44(2): 117–121.

Chizhikov VE, Spiropoulou CF, Morzunov SP, Monroe MC, Peters CJ, Nichol ST. Complete genetic characterization and analysis of isolation of Sin Nombre virus. J Virol 1995; 69(12): 8132–8136.

Cho HW, Howard CR. Antibody responses in humans to an inactivated hantavirus vaccine (Hantavax). Vaccine 1999; 17(20–21): 2569–2575.

Clegg JC. Molecular phylogeny of the arenaviruses. Curr Top Microbiol Immunol 2002; 262: 1–24.

Clegg JCS, Lloyd G. The African arenaviruses Lassa and Mopeia: biological and immuno-chemical comparisons, Segmented Negative Strand Viruses. Orlando: Academic Press, 1984, pp. 341–347.

Close WT. Documentary Novel of its First Explosion. New York: Ivy Books; 1995.

Committee to Study Priorities for Vaccine Development. Vaccines for the 21st Century: A Tool for Decisionmaking. Washington, DC: National Academy Press, 2000.

Corver J, Ortiz A, Allison SL, Schalich J, Heinz FX, Wilschut J. Membrane fusion activity of tick-borne encephalitis virus and recombinant subviral particles in a liposomal model system. Virology 2000; 269(1): 37–46.

Dandawate CN, Desai GB, Achar TR, Banerjee K. Field evaluation of formalin inactivated Kyasanur forest disease virus tissue culture vaccine in three districts of Karnataka state. Indian J Med Res 1994; 99: 152–158.

Davies FG, Linthicum KJ, James AD. Rainfall and epizootic Rift Valley fever. Bull World Health Organ 1985; 63(5): 941–943.

de Manzione N, Salas RA, Paredes H, Godoy O, Rojas L, Araoz F, Fulhorst CF, Ksiazek TG, Mills JN, Ellis BA, Peters CJ, Tesh RB. Venezuelan hemorrhagic fever: clinical and epidemiological studies of 165 cases. Clin Infect Dis 1998; 26(2): 308–313.

Dessen A, Volchkov V, Dolnik O, Klenk HD, Weissenhorn W. Crystal structure of the matrix protein VP40 from Ebola virus. EMBO J 2000; 19(16): 4228–4236.

Diamond J. Guns, Germs and Steel. London: Jonathan Cape; 1997.

Djavani M, Yin C, Lukashevich IS, Rodas J, Rai SK, Salvato MS. Mucosal immunization with *Salmonella typhimurium* expressing Lassa virus nucleocapsid protein cross-protects mice from lethal challenge with lymphocytic choriomeningitis virus. J Hum Virol 2001; 4(2): 103–108.

Dowell SF, Mukunu R, Ksiazek TG, Khan AS, Rollin PE, Peters CJ. Transmission of Ebola hemorrhagic fever: a study of risk factors in family members, Kikwit, Democratic Republic of the Congo, 1995. Commission de Lutte contre les Epidemies a Kikwit. J Infect Dis 1999; 179(Suppl 1): S87–S91.

Drosten C, Gottig S, Schilling S, Asper M, Panning M, Schmitz H, Gunther S. Rapid detection and quantification of RNA of Ebola and Marburg viruses, Lassa virus, Crimean-Congo hemorrhagic fever virus, Rift Valley fever virus, dengue virus, and yellow fever virus by real-time reverse transcription-PCR. J Clin Microbiol 2002; 40(7): 2323–2330.

Durbin AP, Karron RA, Sun W, Vaughn DW, Reynolds MJ, Perreault JR, Thumar B, Men R, Lai CJ, Elkins WR, Chanock RM, Murphy BR, Whitehead SS. Attenuation and immunogenicity in humans of a live dengue virus type-4 vaccine candidate with a 30 nucleotide deletion in its 3'-untranslated region. Am J Trop Med Hyg 2001; 65(5): 405–413.

Dyer A. The English sweating sickness of 1551: an epidemic anatomized. Med Hist 1997; 41: 362–384.

Earle DP. Analysis of sequential physiologic derangements in epidemic hemorrhagic fever; with a commentary on management. Am J Med 1954; 16(5): 690–709.

Eddy GA, Peters CJ. The extended horizons of Rift Valley fever: current and projected immunogens. Prog Clin Biol Res 1980; 47: 179–191.

Elliott LH, Kiley MP, McCormick JB. Descriptive analysis of Ebola virus proteins. Virology 1985; 147(1): 169–176.

Ellis DS, Simpson IH, Francis DP, Knobloch J, Bowen ET, Lolik P, Deng IM. Ultrastructure of Ebola virus particles in human liver. J Clin Pathol 1978; 31(3): 201–208.

Ellis DS, Stamford S, Lloyd G, Bowen ET, Platt GS, Way H, Simpson DI. Ebola and Marburg viruses: I. Some ultrastructural differences between strains when grown in Vero cells. J Med Virol 1979; 4(3): 201–211.

Enria DA, Briggiler AM, Fernandez NJ, Levis SC, Maiztegui JI. Importance of dose of neutralising antibodies in treatment of Argentine haemorrhagic fever with immune plasma. Lancet 1984; 2(8397): 255–256.

Feldmann H, Nichol ST, Klenk HD, Peters CJ, Sanchez A. Characterization of filoviruses based on differences in structure and antigenicity of the virion glycoprotein. Virology 1994; 199(2): 469–473.

Feldmann H, Bugany H, Mahner F, Klenk HD, Drenckhahn D, Schnittler HJ. Filovirus-induced endothelial leakage triggered by infected monocytes/macrophages. J Virol 1996; 70(4): 2208–2214.

Feldmann H, Volchkov V, Volchkova V, Stroher U, Klenk HD. Biosynthesis and role of filoviral glycoproteins. J Gen Virol 2001; 82: 2839–2848.

Feldmann H, Jones S, Klenk HD, Schnittler HJ. Ebola virus: from discovery to vaccine. Nat Rev Immunol 2003; 3(8): 677–685.

Fisher-Hoch SP. Arenavirus pathophysiology. In: The Arenaviridae (Salvato MS, editor). New York: Plenum Press; 1993; pp. 299–323.

Fisher-Hoch SP, Mitchell SW, Sasso DR, Lange JV, Ramsey R, McCormick JB. Physiological and immunologic disturbances associated with shock in a primate model of Lassa fever. J Infect Dis 1987; 155(3): 465–474.

Fisher-Hoch SP, Perez-Oronoz GI, Jackson EL, Hermann LM, Brown BG. Filovirus clearance in non-human primates. Lancet 1992; 340(8817): 451–453.

Fisher-Hoch SP, Hutwagner L, Brown B, McCormick JB. Effective vaccine for Lassa fever. J Virol 2000; 74(15): 6777–6783.

Flamand M, Megret F, Mathieu M, Lepault J, Rey FA, Deubel V. Dengue virus type 1 nonstructural glycoprotein NS1 is secreted from mammalian cells as a soluble hexamer in a glycosylation-dependent fashion. J Virol 1999; 73(7): 6104–6110.

Fonseca BA, Pincus S, Shope RE, Paoletti E, Mason PW. Recombinant vaccinia viruses co-expressing dengue-1 glycoproteins prM and E induce neutralizing antibodies in mice. Vaccine 1994; 12(3): 279–285.

Formenty P, Hatz C, Le Guenno B, Stoll A, Rogenmoser P, Widmer A. Human infection due to Ebola virus, subtype Cote d'Ivoire: clinical and biologic presentation. J Infect Dis 1999; 179(Suppl 1): S48–S53.

Fulhorst CF, Bowen MD, Ksiazek TG, Rollin PE, Nichol ST, Kosoy MY, Peters CJ. Isolation and characterization of Whitewater Arroyo virus, a novel North American arenavirus. Virology 1996; 224(1): 114–120.

Fuller-Pace F, Southern P. Detection of virus-specific RNA-dependent RNA polymerase activity in extracts from cells infected with lymphocytic choriomeningitis virus: in vitro synthesis of full-length viral RNA species. J Virol 1989; 63: 1938–1944.

Gajdusek DC. Virus hemorrhagic fevers. Special reference to hemorrhagic fever with renal syndrome (epidemic hemorrhagic fever). J Pediatr 1962; 60: 841–857.

Garcia JB, Morzunov SP, Levis S, Rowe J, Calderon G, Enria D, Sabattini M, Buchmeier MJ, Bowen MD, St Jeor SC. Genetic diversity of the Junin virus in Argentina: geographic and temporal patterns. Virology 2000; 272(1): 127–136.

Garcin D, Kolakofsky D. Tacaribe arenavirus RNA synthesis in vitro is primer dependent and suggests an unusual model for the initiation of genome replication. J Virol 1992; 66(3): 1370–1376.

Gavrilovskaya IN, Brown EJ, Ginsberg MH, Mackow ER. Cellular entry of hantaviruses which cause hemorrhagic fever with renal syndrome is mediated by beta3 integrins. J Virol 1999; 73(5): 3951–3959.

Gear JS, Cassel GA, Gear AJ, Trappler B, Clausen L, Meyers AM, Kew MC, Bothwell TH, Sher R, Miller GB, Schneider J, Koornhof HJ, Gomperts ED, Isaacson M, Gear JH. Outbreak of Marburg virus disease in Johannesburg. Br Med J 1975; 4(5995): 489–493.

Geisbert TW, Jahrling PB. Use of immunoelectron microscopy to show Ebola virus during the 1989 United States epizootic. J Clin Pathol 1990; 43(10): 813–816.

Georges-Courbot MC, Sanchez A, Lu CY, Baize S, Leroy E, Lansout-Soukate J, Tevi-Benissan C, Georges AJ, Trappier SG, Zaki SR, Swanepoel R, Leman PA, Rollin PE, Peters CJ, Nichol ST, Ksiazek TG. Isolation and phylogenetic characterization of Ebola viruses causing different outbreaks in Gabon. Emerg Infect Dis 1997; 3(1): 59–62.

Glass GE, Yates TL, Fine JB, Shields TM, Kendall JB, Hope AG, Parmenter CA, Peters CJ, Ksiazek TG, Li CS, Patz JA, Mills JN. Satellite imagery characterizes local animal reservoir populations of Sin Nombre virus in the southwestern United States. Proc Natl Acad Sci USA 2002; 99(26): 16817–16822.

Gonzalez JP, Josse R, Johnson ED, Merlin M, Georges AJ, Abandja J, Danyod M, Delaporte E, Dupont A, Ghogomu A. Antibody prevalence against haemorrhagic fever viruses in randomized representative Central African populations. Res Virol 1989; 140(4): 319–331.

Gonzalez JP, Nakoune E, Slenczka W, Vidal P, Morvan JM. Ebola and Marburg virus antibody prevalence in selected populations of the Central African Republic. Microbes Infect 2000; 2(1): 39–44.

Groen J, Gerding MN, Jordans JG, Clement JP, Nieuwenhuijs JH, Osterhaus AD. Hantavirus infections in The Netherlands: epidemiology and disease. Epidemiol Infect 1995; 114(2): 373–383.

Gubler DJ. The global pandemic of dengue/dengue haemorrhagic fever: current status and prospects for the future. Ann Acad Med Singapore 1998; 27(2): 227–234.

Gubler DJ. Epidemic dengue/dengue hemorrhagic fever as a public health, social and economic problem in the 21st century. Trends Microbiol 2002; 10(2): 100–103.

Guirakhoo F, Arroyo J, Pugachev KV, Miller C, Zhang ZX, Weltzin R, Georgakopoulos K, Catalan J, Ocran S, Soike K, Ratterree M, Monath TP. Construction, safety, and immunogenicity in nonhuman primates of a chimeric yellow fever-dengue virus tetravalent vaccine. J Virol 2001; 75(16): 7290–7304.

Guirakhoo F, Pugachev K, Arroyo J, Miller C, Zhang ZX, Weltzin R, Georgakopoulos K, Catalan J, Ocran S, Draper K, Monath TP. Viremia and immunogenicity in nonhuman primates of a tetravalent yellow fever-dengue chimeric vaccine: genetic reconstructions, dose adjustment, and antibody responses against wild-type dengue virus isolates. Virology 2002; 298(1): 146–159.

Gunther S, Emmerich P, Laue T, Kuhle O, Asper M, Jung A, Grewing T, ter Meulen J, Schmitz H. Imported Lassa fever in Germany: molecular characterization of a new Lassa virus strain. Emerg Infect Dis 2000; 6(5): 466–476.

Gupta M, Mahanty S, Bray M, Ahmed R, Rollin PE. Passive transfer of antibodies protects immunocompetent and imunodeficient mice against lethal Ebola virus infection without complete inhibition of viral replication. J Virol 2001; 75(10): 4649–4654.

Hallin GW, Simpson SQ, Crowell RE, James DS, Koster FT, Mertz GJ, Levy H. Cardiopulmonary manifestations of hantavirus pulmonary syndrome. Crit Care Med 1996; 24(2): 252–258.

Halstead SB, O'Rourke EJ. Dengue viruses and mononuclear phagocytes. I. Infection enhancement by non-neutralizing antibody. J Exp Med 1977; 146(1): 201–217.

Hannon GJ. RNA interference. Nature 2002; 418(6894): 244–251.

Harrington DG, Lupton HW, Crabbs CL, Peters CJ, Reynolds JA, Slone TW Jr. Evaluation of a formalin-inactivated Rift Valley fever vaccine in sheep. Am J Vet Res 1980; 41(10): 1559–1564.

Hefti HP, Frese M, Landis H, Di Paolo C, Aguzzi A, Haller O, Pavlovic J. Human MxA protein protects mice lacking a functional alpha/beta interferon system against La crosse virus and other lethal viral infections. J Virol 1999; 73(8): 6984–6991.

Hevey M, Negley D, Pushko P, Smith J, Schmaljohn A. Marburg virus vaccines based upon alphavirus replicons protect guinea pigs and nonhuman primates. Virology 1998; 251(1): 28–37.

Hevey M, Negley D, Schmaljohn A. Characterization of monoclonal antibodies to Marburg virus (strain Musoke) glycoprotein and identification of two protective epitopes. Virology 2003; 314(1): 350–357.

Heymann DL, Rodier GR. Hot spots in a wired world: WHO surveillance of emerging and re-emerging infectious diseases. Lancet Infect Dis 2001; 1(5): 345–353.

Heymann DL, Weisfeld JS, Webb PA, Johnson KM, Cairns T, Berquist H. Ebola hemorrhagic fever: Tandala, Zaire, 1977–1978. J Infect Dis 1980; 142(3): 372–376.

Hjelle B, Yates T. Modeling hantavirus maintenance and transmission in rodent communities. Curr Top Microbiol Immunol 2001; 256: 77–90.

Hjelle B, Jenison S, Torrez-Martinez N, Herring B, Quan S, Polito A, Pichuantes S, Yamada T, Morris C, Elgh F, Lee HW, Artsob H, Dinello R. Rapid and specific detection of Sin Nombre virus antibodies in patients with hantavirus pulmonary syndrome by a strip immunoblot assay suitable for field diagnosis. J Clin Microbiol 1997; 35(3): 600–608.

Holmes FF. Anne Boleyn, the sweating sickness, and the hantavirus: a review of an old disease with a modern interpretation. J Med Biogr 1998; 6(1): 43–48.

Honig JE, Osborne JC, Nichol ST. Crimean-Congo hemorrhagic fever virus genome L RNA segment and encoded protein. Virology 2004a; 321(1): 29–35.

Honig JE, Osborne JC, Nichol ST. The high genetic variation of viruses of the genus *Nairovirus* reflects the diversity of their predominant tick hosts. Virology 2004b; 318(1): 10–16.

Hooper JW, Larsen T, Custer DM, Schmaljohn CS. A lethal disease model for hantavirus pulmonary syndrome. Virology 2001; 289(1): 6–14.

Howard CR. Arenaviruses. In: Perspectives in Medical Virology (Zuckerman AJ, editor). vol. 2. Amsterdam: Elsevier; 1986.

Huang C, Jin B, Wang M, Li E, Sun C. Hemorrhagic fever with renal syndrome: relationship between pathogenesis and cellular immunity. J Infect Dis 1994; 169(4): 868–870.

Huang CY, Butrapet S, Pierro DJ, Chang GJ, Hunt AR, Bhamarapravati N, Gubler DJ, Kinney RM. Chimeric dengue type 2 (vaccine strain PDK-53)/dengue type 1 virus as a potential candidate dengue type 1 virus vaccine. J Virol 2000; 74(7): 3020–3028.

Huggins JW. Prospects for treatment of viral hemorrhagic fevers with ribavirin, a broad-spectrum antiviral drug. Rev Infect Dis 1989; 11(Suppl 4): S750–S761.

Huggins JW, Hsiang CM, Cosgriff TM, Guang MY, Smith JI, Wu ZO, LeDuc JW, Zheng ZM, Meegan JM, Wang QN. Prospective, double-blind, concurrent, placebo-controlled clinical trial of intravenous ribavirin therapy of hemorrhagic fever with renal syndrome. J Infect Dis 1991; 164(6): 1119–1127.

Hujakka H, Koistinen V, Kuronen I, Eerikainen P, Parviainen M, Lundkvist A, Vaheri A, Vapalahti O, Narvanen A. Diagnostic rapid tests for acute hantavirus infections: specific tests for Hantaan, Dobrava and Puumala viruses versus a hantavirus combination test. J Virol Methods 2003; 108(1): 117–122.

Humphreys M. Dengue fever: Breakbone fever. In: Plague, Pox and Pestilence: Disease in History (Kiple KF, editor). London: Weidenfeld & Nicolson; 1997; pp. 92–97.

Hung SL, Lee PL, Chen HW, Chen LK, Kao CL, King CC. Analysis of the steps involved in Dengue virus entry into host cells. Virology 1999; 257(1): 156–167.

Ibrahim MS, Turell MJ, Knauert FK, Lofts RS. Detection of Rift Valley fever virus in mosquitoes by RT-PCR. Mol Cell Probes 1997; 11(1): 49–53.

Ishak R, Tovey DG, Howard CR. Morphogenesis of yellow fever virus 17D in infected cell cultures. J Gen Virol 1988; 69(Pt 2): 325–335.

Jacamo R, Lopez N, Wilda M, Franze-Fernandez MT. Tacaribe virus Z protein interacts with the L polymerase protein to inhibit viral RNA synthesis. J Virol 2003; 77(19): 10383–10393.

Jacobs MG, Robinson PJ, Bletchly C, Mackenzie JM, Young PR. Dengue virus nonstructural protein 1 is expressed in a glycosyl-phosphatidylinositol-linked form that is capable of signal transduction. FASEB J 2000; 14(11): 1603–1610.

Jahrling PB, Geisbert TW, Geisbert JB, Swearengen JR, Bray M, Jaax NK, Huggins JW, LeDuc JW, Peters CJ. Evaluation of immune globulin and recombinant interferon-alpha2b for treatment of experimental Ebola virus infections. J Infect Dis 1999; 179(Suppl 1): S224–S234.

Jennings AD, Gibson CA, Miller BR, Mathews JH, Mitchell CJ, Roehrig JT, Wood DJ, Taffs F, Sil BK, Whitby SN. Analysis of a yellow fever virus isolated from a fatal case of vaccine-associated human encephalitis. J Infect Dis 1994; 169(3): 512–518.

Johansson M, Brooks AJ, Jans DA, Vasudevan SG. A small region of the dengue virus-encoded RNA-dependent RNA polymerase, NS5, confers interaction with both the nuclear transport receptor importin-beta and the viral helicase, NS3. J Gen Virol 2001; 82(Pt 4): 735–745.

Johnson AJ, Roehrig JT. New mouse model for dengue virus vaccine testing. J Virol 1999; 73(1): 783–786.

Johnson KM, Webb PA, Justines G. Biology of Tacaribe-complex virus. In: Lymphocytic Choriomeningitis virus and other Arenaviruses (Lehmann-Grube F, editor). Vienna: Springer; 1973; pp. 241–258.

Johnson BK, Ocheng D, Gitau LG, Gichogo A, Tukei PM, Ngindu A, Langatt A, Smith DH, Johnson KM, Kiley MP, Swanepoel R, Isaacson M. Viral haemorrhagic fever surveillance in Kenya, 1980–1981. Trop Geogr Med 1983; 35(1): 43–47.

Johnson KM, McCormick JB, Webb PA, Smith ES, Elliott LH, King IJ. Clinical virology of Lassa fever in hospitalized patients. J Infect Dis 1987; 155(3): 456–464.

Johnson ED, Johnson BK, Silverstein D, Tukei P, Geisbert TW, Sanchez AN, Jahrling PB. Characterization of a new Marburg virus isolated from a 1987 fatal case in Kenya. Arch Virol Suppl 1996; 11: 101–114.

Kane A, Lloyd J, Zaffran M, Simonsen L, Kane M. Transmission of hepatitis B, hepatitis C and human immunodeficiency viruses through unsafe injections in the developing world: model-based regional estimates. Bull World Health Organ 1999; 77(10): 801–807.

Kanerva M, Vaheri A, Mustonen J, Partanen J. High-producer allele of tumour necrosis factor-alpha is part of the susceptibility MHC haplotype in severe puumala virus-induced nephropathia epidemica. Scand J Infect Dis 1998; 30(5): 532–534.

Kanesa-Thasan N. Development of dengue vaccines: an overview. Indian Pediatr 1998; 35(2): 97–100.

Kanesa-Thasan N, Sun W, Kim-Ahn G, Van Albert S, Putnak JR, King A, Raengsakulsrach B, Christ-Schmidt H, Gilson K, Zahradnik JM, Vaughn DW, Innis BL, Saluzzo JF, Hoke CH Jr. Safety and immunogenicity of attenuated dengue virus vaccines (Aventis Pasteur) in human volunteers. Vaccine 2001; 19(23–24): 3179–3188.

Kark JD, Aynor Y, Peters CJ. A Rift Valley fever vaccine trial. I. Side effects and serologic response over a six-month follow-up. Am J Epidemiol 1982; 116(5): 808–820.

Kark JD, Aynor Y, Peters CJ. A Rift Valley fever vaccine trial: 2. Serological response to booster doses with a comparison of intradermal versus subcutaneous injection. Vaccine 1985; 3(2): 117–122.

Kilgore PE, Ksiazek TG, Rollin PE, Mills JN, Villagra MR, Montenegro MJ, Costales MA, Paredes LC, Peters CJ. Treatment of Bolivian hemorrhagic fever with intravenous ribavirin. Clin Infect Dis 1997; 24(4): 718–722.

Kinney RM, Huang CY. Development of new vaccines against dengue fever and Japanese encephalitis. Intervirology 2001; 44(2–3): 176–197.

Kinsella E, Martin SG, Grolla A, Czub M, Feldmann H, Flick R. Sequence determination of the Crimean-Congo hemorrhagic fever virus L segment. Virology 2004; 321(1): 23–28.

Klenerman P, Hengartner H, Zinkernagel RM. A non-retroviral RNA virus persists in DNA form. Nature 1997; 390: 298–301.

Klenk HD, Rott R. The molecular biology of influenza virus pathogenicity. Adv Virus Res 1988; 34: 247–281.

Kochel TJ, Watts DM, Halstead SB, Hayes CG, Espinoza A, Felices V, Caceda R, Bautista CT, Montoya Y, Douglas S, Russell KL. Effect of dengue-1 antibodies on American dengue-2 viral infection and dengue haemorrhagic fever. Lancet 2002; 360(9329): 310–312.

Kochs G, Janzen C, Hohenberg H, Haller O. Antivirally active MxA protein sequesters La Crosse virus nucleocapsid protein into perinuclear complexes. Proc Natl Acad Sci USA 2002; 99(5): 3153–3158.

Kosoy MY, Elliott LH, Ksiazek TG, Fulhorst CF, Rollin PE, Childs JE, Mills JN, Maupin GO, Peters CJ. Prevalence of antibodies to arenaviruses in rodents from the southern and western United States: evidence for an arenavirus associated with the genus *Neotoma*. Am J Trop Med Hyg 1996; 54(6): 570–576.

Ksiazek TG, Rollin PE, Jahrling PB, Johnson E, Dalgard DW, Peters CJ. Enzyme immunosorbent assay for Ebola virus antigens in tissues of infected primates. J Clin Microbiol 1992; 30(4): 947–950.

Kuhn RJ, Zhang W, Rossmann MG, Pletnev SV, Corver J, Lenches E, Jones CT, Mukhopadhyay S, Chipman PR, Strauss EG, Baker TS, Strauss JH. Structure of dengue virus: implications for flavivirus organization, maturation, and fusion. Cell 2002; 108(5): 717–725.

Kummerer BM, Rice CM. Mutations in the yellow fever virus nonstructural protein NS2A selectively block production of infectious particles. J Virol 2002; 76(10): 4773–4784.

Kurane I, Takasaki T. Dengue fever and dengue haemorrhagic fever: challenges of controlling an enemy still at large. Rev Med Virol 2001; 11(5): 301–311.

Lau LL, Jamieson BD, Somasundaram T, Ahmed R. Cytotoxic T-cell memory without antigen. Nature 1994; 369(6482): 648–652.

Le May N, Dubaele S, De Santis LP, Billecocq A, Bouloy M, Egly JM. TFIIH transcription factor, a target for the Rift Valley hemorrhagic fever virus. Cell 2004; 116(4): 541–550.

Lee HW, van der GG. Hemorrhagic fever with renal syndrome. Prog Med Virol 1989; 36: 62–102.

Lehmann-Grube F. Lymphocytic choriomeningitis virus. Virol Monogr 1971; 10: 1.

Lenz O, ter Meulen J, Klenk HD, Seidah NG, Garten W. The Lassa virus glycoprotein precursor GP-C is proteolytically processed by subtilase SKI-1/S1P. Proc Natl Acad Sci USA 2001; 98(22): 12701–12705.

Levis SC, Saavedra MC. Endogenous interferon in Argentine haemorrhagic fever. J Infect Dis 1984; 149: 428–433.

Li H, Clum S, You S, Ebner KE, Padmanabhan R. The serine protease and RNA-stimulated nucleoside triphosphatase and RNA helicase functional domains of dengue virus type 2 NS3 converge within a region of 20 amino acids. J Virol 1999; 73(4): 3108–3116.

Lin D, Li L, Dick D, Shope RE, Feldmann H, Barrett AD, Holbrook MR. Analysis of the complete genome of the tick-borne flavivirus Omsk hemorrhagic fever virus. Virology 2003; 313(1): 81–90.

Lindenbach BD, Rice CM. Trans-Complementation of yellow fever virus NS1 reveals a role in early RNA replication. J Virol 1997; 71(12): 9608–9617.

Lindenbach BD, Rice CM. Genetic interaction of flavivirus nonstructural proteins NS1 and NS4A as a determinant of replicase function. J Virol 1999; 73(6): 4611–4621.

Linderholm M, Ahlm C, Settergren B, Waage A, Tarnvik A. Elevated plasma levels of tumor necrosis factor (TNF)-alpha, soluble TNF receptors, interleukin (IL)-6, and IL-10 in patients with hemorrhagic fever with renal syndrome. J Infect Dis 1996; 173(1): 38–43.

Linthicum KJ, Davies FG, Kairo A, Bailey CL. Rift Valley fever virus (family Bunyaviridae, genus *Phlebovirus*). Isolations from Diptera collected during an inter-epizootic period in Kenya. J Hyg (Lond) 1985; 95(1): 197–209.

Linthicum KJ, Anyamba A, Tucker CJ, Kelley PW, Myers MF, Peters CJ. Climate and satellite indicators to forecast Rift Valley fever epidemics in Kenya. Science 1999; 285(5426): 397–400.

Lisieux T, Coimbra M, Nassar ES, Burattini MN, de Souza LT, Ferreira I, Rocco IM, da Rosa AP, Vasconcelos PF, Pinheiro FP. New arenavirus isolated in Brazil. Lancet 1994; 343(8894): 391–392.

Lledo L, Gegundez MI, Saz JV, Bahamontes N, Beltran M. Lymphocytic choriomeningitis virus infection in a province of Spain: analysis of sera from the general population and wild rodents. J Med Virol 2003; 70(2): 273–275.

Lopez N, Jacamo R, Franze-Fernandez MT. Transcription and RNA replication of tacaribe virus genome and antigenome analogs require N and L proteins: Z protein is an inhibitor of these processes. J Virol 2001; 75(24): 12241–12251.

Lorenz IC, Allison SL, Heinz FX, Helenius A. Folding and dimerization of tick-borne encephalitis virus envelope proteins prM and E in the endoplasmic reticulum. J Virol 2002; 76(11): 5480–5491.

Lozano ME, Enria D, Maiztegui JI, Grau O, Romanowski V. Rapid diagnosis of Argentine hemorrhagic fever by reverse transcriptase PCR-based assay. J Clin Microbiol 1995; 33(5): 1327–1332.

Lu Q, Zhu Z, Weng J. Immune responses to inactivated vaccine in people naturally infected with hantaviruses. J Med Virol 1996; 49(4): 333–335.

Lukashevich IS, Djavani M, Shapiro K, Sanchez A, Ravkov E, Nichol ST, Salvato MS. The Lassa fever virus L gene: nucleotide sequence, comparison, and precipitation of a predicted 250 kDa protein with monospecific antiserum. J Gen Virol 1997; 78(Pt 3): 547–551.

Maiztegui JI, Fernandez JM, de Damilano AJ. Efficacy of immune plasma in treatment of Argentine haemorrhagic fever and association between infection and a late neurological syndrome. Lancet 1979; ii: 1216–1217.

Maiztegui JI, Feuillade M, Briggiler A. Progressive extension of the endemic area and changing incidence of Argentine hemorrhagic fever. Med Microbiol Immunol (Berl) 1986; 175(2–3): 149–152.

Maiztegui JI, McKee KT Jr, Barrera Oro JG, Harrison LH, Gibbs PH, Feuillade MR, Enria DA, Briggiler AM, Levis SC, Ambrosio AM, Halsey NA, Peters CJ. Protective efficacy of a live attenuated vaccine against Argentine hemorrhagic fever. AHF Study Group. J Infect Dis 1998; 177(2): 277–283.

Malashkevich VN, Schneider BJ, McNally ML, Milhollen MA, Pang JX, Kim PS. Core structure of the envelope glycoprotein GP2 from Ebola virus at 1.9-A resolution. Proc Natl Acad Sci USA 1999; 96(6): 2662–2667.

Manns MP, McHutchison JG, Gordon SC, Rustgi VK, Shiffman M, Reindollar R, Goodman ZD, Koury K, Ling M, Albrecht JK. Peginterferon alfa-2b plus ribavirin compared with interferon alfa-2b plus ribavirin for initial treatment of chronic hepatitis C: a randomised trial. Lancet 2001; 358(9286): 958–965.

Marianneau P, Megret F, Olivier R, Morens DM, Deubel V. Dengue 1 virus binding to human hepatoma HepG2 and simian Vero cell surfaces differs. J Gen Virol 1996; 77(Pt 10): 2547–2554.

Marr JS, Kiracofe JB. Was the huey cocoliztli a haemorrhagic fever? Med Hist 2000; 44(3): 341–362.

Markoff L, Pang X, Houng Hs HS, Falgout B, Olsen R, Jones E, Polo S. Derivation and characterization of a dengue type 1 host range-restricted mutant virus that is attenuated and highly immunogenic in monkeys. J Virol 2002; 76(7): 3318–3328.

Marrie TJ, Saron MF. Seroprevalence of lymphocytic choriomeningitis virus in Nova Scotia. Am J Trop Med Hyg 1998; 58(1): 47–49.

Martini GA. Marburg virus disease. Postgrad Med J 1973; 49(574): 542–546.

Martini GA, Siegert R. Marburg Virus Disease. Berlin: Springer; 1971.

Maruyama T, Parren PW, Sanchez A, Rensink I, Rodriguez LL, Khan AS, Peters CJ, Burton DR. Recombinant human monoclonal antibodies to Ebola virus. J Infect Dis 1999a; 179(Suppl 1): S235–S239.

Maruyama T, Rodriguez LL, Jahrling PB, Sanchez A, Khan AS, Nichol ST, Peters CJ, Parren PW, Burton DR. Ebola virus can be effectively neutralized by antibody produced in natural human infection. J Virol 1999b; 73(7): 6024–6030.

McClain DJ, Summers PL, Harrison SA, Schmaljohn AL, Schmaljohn CS. Clinical evaluation of a vaccinia-vectored Hantaan virus vaccine. J Med Virol 2000; 60(1): 77–85.

McCormick JB, King IJ, Webb PA, Scribner CL, Craven RB, Johnson KM, Elliott LH, Belmont-Williams R. Lassa fever. Effective therapy with ribavirin. N Engl J Med 1986a; 314(1): 20–26.

McCormick JB, Walker DH, King IJ, Webb PA, Elliott LH, Whitfield SG, Johnson KM. Lassa virus hepatitis: a study of fatal Lassa fever in humans. Am J Trop Med Hyg 1986b; 35(2): 401–407.

McCormick JB, Walker DH, King IJ, Webb PA, Elliott LH, Whitfield SG, Johnson KM. Lassa virus hepatitis: a study of fatal Lassa fever in humans. Am J Trop Med Hyg 1986c; 35(2): 401–407.

McCormick JB, King IJ, Webb PA, Johnson KM, O'Sullivan R, Smith ES, Trippel S, Tong TC. A case-control study of the clinical diagnosis and course of Lassa fever. J Infect Dis 1987a; 155(3): 445–455.

McCormick JB, King IJ, Webb PA, Johnson KM, O'Sullivan R, Smith ES, Trippel S, Tong TC. A case-control study of the clinical diagnosis and course of Lassa fever. J Infect Dis 1987b; 155(3): 445–455.

McCormick JB, Webb PA, Krebs JW, Johnson KM, Smith ES. A prospective study of the epidemiology and ecology of Lassa fever. J Infect Dis 1987c; 155(3): 437–444.

McKee KT Jr, Oro JG, Kuehne AI, Spisso JA, Mahlandt BG. Safety and immunogenicity of a live-attenuated Junin (Argentine hemorrhagic fever) vaccine in rhesus macaques. Am J Trop Med Hyg 1993; 48(3): 403–411.

Meegan JM. The Rift Valley fever epizootic in Egypt 1977–78. 1. Description of the epizootic and virological studies. Trans R Soc Trop Med Hyg 1979; 73(6): 618–623.

Meers PD. Yellow fever in Swansea, 1865. J Hyg (Lond) 1986; 97(1): 185–191.

Meissner F, Maruyama T, Frentsch M, Hessell AJ, Rodriguez LL, Geisbert TW, Jahrling PB, Burton DR, Parren PW. Detection of antibodies against the four subtypes of Ebola virus in sera from any species using a novel antibody-phage indicator assay. Virology 2002; 300(2): 236–243.

Men R, Bray M, Lai CJ. Carboxy-terminally truncated dengue virus envelope glycoproteins expressed on the cell surface and secreted extracellularly exhibit increased immunogenicity in mice. J Virol 1991; 65(3): 1400–1407.

Men R, Bray M, Clark D, Chanock RM, Lai CJ. Dengue type 4 virus mutants containing deletions in the 3′ noncoding region of the RNA genome: analysis of growth restriction in cell culture and altered viremia pattern and immunogenicity in rhesus monkeys. J Virol 1996; 70(6): 3930–3937.

Mills JN, Barrera-Oro JG, Bressler DS, Childs JE, Tesh RB, Smith JF, Enria DA, Geisbert TW, McKee KT Jr, Bowen MD, Peters CJ, Jahrling PB. Characterization of Oliveros virus, a new member of the Tacaribe complex (Arenaviridae: Arenavirus). Am J Trop Med Hyg 1996; 54(4): 399–404.

Mitchell SW, McCormick JB. Physicochemical inactivation of Lassa, Ebola, and Marburg viruses and effect on clinical laboratory analyses. J Clin Microbiol 1984; 20(3): 486–489.

Modis Y, Ogata S, Clements D, Harrison SC. A ligand-binding pocket in the dengue virus envelope glycoprotein. Proc Natl Acad Sci USA 2003; 100(12): 6986–6991.

Modis Y, Ogata S, Clements D, Harrison SC. Structure of the dengue virus envelope protein after membrane fusion. Nature 2004; 427(6972): 313–319.

Monath TP. (1985) Socioeconomic impact of arbovirus diseases—a world view, Proceedings of the 4th symposium on Arbovirus Research in Australia. pp. 3–15.

Monath TP. Lassa fever—new issues raised by field studies in West Africa. J Infect Dis 1987; 155(3): 433–436.

Monath TP. Ecology of Marburg and Ebola viruses: speculations and directions for future research. J Infect Dis 1999; 179(Suppl 1): S127–S138.

Monath TP. Yellow fever: an update. Lancet Infect Dis 2001; 1(1): 11–20.

Montali RJ, Connolly BM, Armstrong DL, Scanga CA, Holmes KV. Pathology and immunohistochemistry of callitrichid hepatitis, and emerging disease of captive New World primates caused by lymphocytic choriomeningitis virus. Am J Pathol 1995; 147(5): 1441–1449.

Morikawa S, Qing T, Xinqin Z, Saijo M, Kurane I. Genetic diversity of the M RNA segment among Crimean-Congo hemorrhagic fever virus isolates in China. Virology 2002; 296(1): 159–164.

Morrill JC, Jennings GB, Caplen H, Turell MJ, Johnson AJ, Peters CJ. Pathogenicity and immunogenicity of a mutagen-attenuated Rift Valley fever virus immunogen in pregnant ewes. Am J Vet Res 1987; 48(7): 1042–1047.

Morrill JC, Carpenter L, Taylor D, Ramsburg HH, Quance J, Peters CJ. Further evaluation of a mutagen-attenuated Rift Valley fever vaccine in sheep. Vaccine 1991; 9(1): 35–41.

Morrison HG, Bauer SP, Lange JV, Esposito JJ, McCormick JB, Auperin DD. Protection of guinea pigs from Lassa fever by vaccinia virus recombinants expressing the nucleoprotein or the envelope glycoproteins of Lassa virus. Virology 1989; 171(1): 179–188.

Mortimer PP. The control of yellow fever: a centennial account. Microbiol Today 2002; 29: 24–26.

Morvan JM, Deubel V, Gounon P, Nakoune E, Barriere P, Murri S, Perpete O, Selekon B, Coudrier D, Gautier-Hion A, Colyn M, Volehkov V. Identification of Ebola virus sequences present as RNA or DNA in organs of terrestrial small mammals of the Central African Republic. Microbes Infect 1999; 1(14): 1193–1201.

Morzunov SP, Rowe JE, Ksiazek TG, Peters CJ, St Jeor SC, Nichol ST. Genetic analysis of the diversity and origin of hantaviruses in *Peromyscus leucopus* mice in North America. J Virol 1998; 72(1): 57–64.

Muhlberger E, Weik M, Volchkov VE, Klenk HD, Becker S. Comparison of the transcription and replication strategies of Marburg virus and Ebola virus by using artificial replication systems. J Virol 1999; 73(3): 2333–2342.

Mupapa K, Massamba M, Kibadi K, Kuvula K, Bwaka A, Kipasa M, Colebunders R, Muyembe-Tamfum JJ. Treatment of Ebola hemorrhagic fever with blood transfusions from convalescent patients. International Scientific and Technical Committee. J Infect Dis 1999; 179(Suppl 1): S18–S23.

Murali-Krishna K, Lau LL, Sambhara S, Lemonnier F, Altman J, Ahmed R. Persistence of memory CD8 T cells in MHC class I-deficient mice. Science 1999; 286(5443): 1377–1381.

Murphy FA, Whitfield SG. Morphology and morphogenesis of arenaviruses. Bull World Health Organ 1975; 52(4–6): 409–419.

Murphy ME, Kariwa H, Mizutani T, Yoshimatsu K, Arikawa J, Takashima I. In vitro antiviral activity of lactoferrin and ribavirin upon hantavirus. Arch Virol 2000; 145(8): 1571–1582.

Mustonen J, Partanen J, Kanerva M, Pietila K, Vapalahti O, Pasternack A, Vaheri A. Association of HLA B27 with benign clinical course of nephropathia epidemica caused by Puumala hantavirus. Scand J Immunol 1998; 47(3): 277–279.

Nasidi A, Monath TP, Vandenberg J, Tomori O, Calisher CH, Hurtgen X, Munube GR, Sorungbe AO, Okafor GC, Wali S. Yellow fever vaccination and pregnancy: a four-year prospective study. Trans R Soc Trop Med Hyg 1993; 87(3): 337–339.

Navarro-Sanchez E, Altmeyer R, Amara A, Schwartz O, Fieschi F, Virelizier JL, Arenzana-Seisdedos F, Despres P. Dendritic-cell-specific ICAM3-grabbing non-integrin is essential for the productive infection of human dendritic cells by mosquito-cell-derived dengue viruses. EMBO Rep 2003; 4(7): 723–728.

Nemirov K, Vapalahti O, Lundkvist A, Vasilenko V, Golovljova I, Plyusnina A, Niemimaa J, Laakkonen J, Henttonen H, Vaheri A, Plyusnin A. Isolation and characterization of Dobrava hantavirus carried by the striped field mouse (*Apodemus agrarius*) in Estonia. J Gen Virol 1999; 80(Pt 2): 371–379.

Nemirov K, Henttonen H, Vaheri A, Plyusnin A. Phylogenetic evidence for host switching in the evolution of hantaviruses carried by Apodemus mice. Virus Res 2002; 90(1–2): 207–215.

Ni H, Ryman KD, Wang H, Saeed MF, Hull R, Wood D, Minor PD, Watowich SJ, Barrett AD. Interaction of yellow fever virus French neurotropic vaccine strain with monkey brain: characterization of monkey brain membrane receptor escape variants. J Virol 2000; 74(6): 2903–2906.

Nichol S. Bunyaviruses. In: Fields Virology (Knipe D, Howley P, editors). 4th ed. Philadelphia: Lippincott, Williams & Wilkins; 2001; pp. 1603–1633.

Nolte KB, Feddersen RM, Foucar K, Zaki SR, Koster FT, Madar D, Merlin TL, McFeeley PJ, Umland ET, Zumwalt RE. Hantavirus pulmonary syndrome in the United States: a pathological description of a disease caused by a new agent. Hum Pathol 1995; 26(1): 110–120.

Oldstone MB. Arenaviruses. I. The epidemiology molecular and cell biology of arenaviruses. Introduction. Curr Top Microbiol Immunol 2002a; 262: V–XII.

Oldstone MB. Arenaviruses. II. The molecular pathogenesis of arenavirus infections. Introduction. Curr Top Microbiol Immunol 2002b; 263: V–XII.

Padula PJ, Colavecchia SB, Martinez VP, Gonzalez DV, Edelstein A, Miguel SD, Russi J, Riquelme JM, Colucci N, Almiron M, Rabinovich RD. Genetic diversity, distribution, and serological features of hantavirus infection in five countries in South America. J Clin Microbiol 2000a; 38(8): 3029–3035.

Padula PJ, Rossi CM, Della Valle MO, Martinez PV, Colavecchia SB, Edelstein A, Miguel SD, Rabinovich RD, Segura EL. Development and evaluation of a solid-phase enzyme immunoassay based on Andes hantavirus recombinant nucleoprotein. J Med Microbiol 2000b; 49(2): 149–155.

Pattyn SR. Ebola Virus Haemorrhagic Fever. Amsterdam: Elsevier/North Holland Biomedical Press; 1978.

Pavri K. Clinical, clinicopathologic, and hematologic features of Kyasanur Forest disease. Rev Infect Dis 1989; 11(Suppl 4): S854–S859.

Perez M, De La Torre JC. Characterization of the genomic promoter of the prototypic arenavirus lymphocytic choriomeningitis virus. J Virol 2003; 77(2): 1184–1194.

Peters CJ. Hantavirus pulmonary syndrome in the Americas. In: Emerging Infections Volume 2 (Scheld WM, Craig WA, Hughes JM, editors). Washington, DC: ASM Press; 1998; pp. 17–64.

Peters CJ, Khan AS. Hantavirus pulmonary syndrome: the new American hemorrhagic fever. Clin Infect Dis 2002; 34(9): 1224–1231.

Pfau CJ. Biochemical and biophysical properties of the arenaviruses. Prog Med Virol 1974; 18: 64–80.

Pinschewer DD, Perez M, De La Torre JC. Role of the virus nucleoprotein in the regulation of lymphocytic choriomeningitis virus transcription and RNA replication. J Virol 2003; 77(6): 3882–3887.

Pittman PR, Liu CT, Cannon TL, Makuch RS, Mangiafico JA, Gibbs PH, Peters CJ. Immunogenicity of an inactivated Rift Valley fever vaccine in humans: a 12-year experience. Vaccine 1999; 18(1–2): 181–189.

Pletnev AG, Bray M, Huggins J, Lai CJ. Construction and characterization of chimeric tick-borne encephalitis/dengue type 4 viruses. Proc Natl Acad Sci USA 1992; 89(21): 10532–10536.

Plyusnin A. Genetics of hantaviruses: implications to taxonomy. Arch Virol 2002; 147(4): 665–682.

Plyusnin A, Horling J, Kanerva M, Mustonen J, Cheng Y, Partanen J, Vapalahti O, Kukkonen SK, Niemimaa J, Henttonen H, Niklasson B, Lundkvist A, Vaheri A. Puumala hantavirus genome in patients with nephropathia epidemica: correlation of PCR positivity with HLA haplotype and link to viral sequences in local rodents. J Clin Microbiol 1997; 35(5): 1090–1096.

Post PR, Santos CN, Carvalho R, Cruz AC, Rice CM, Galler R. Heterogeneity in envelope protein sequence and N-linked glycosylation among yellow fever virus vaccine strains. Virology 1992; 188(1): 160–167.

Presta L. Antibody engineering for therapeutics. Curr Opin Struct Biol 2003; 13(4): 519–525.

Preston R. The Hot Zone. New York: Random House; 1994.

Pryor MJ, Carr JM, Hocking H, Davidson AD, Li P, Wright PJ. Replication of dengue virus type 2 in human monocyte-derived macrophages: comparisons of isolates and recombinant viruses with substitutions at amino acid 390 in the envelope glycoprotein. Am J Trop Med Hyg 2001; 65(5): 427–434.

Pugachev KV, Guirakhoo F, Trent DW, Monath TP. Traditional and novel approaches to flavivirus vaccines. Int J Parasitol 2003; 33(5–6): 567–582.

Raftery MJ, Kraus AA, Ulrich R, Kruger DH, Schonrich G. Hantavirus infection of dendritic cells. J Virol 2002; 76(21): 10724–10733.

Randall G, Grakoui A, Rice CM. Clearance of replicating hepatitis C virus replicon RNAs in cell culture by small interfering RNAs. Proc Natl Acad Sci USA 2003; 100(1): 235–240.

Rey FA, Heinz FX, Mandl C, Kunz C, Harrison SC. The envelope glycoprotein from tick-borne encephalitis virus at 2 Å resolution. Nature 1995; 375(6529): 291–298.

Reynolds JA, Harrington DG, Crabbs CL, Peters CJ, Di Luzio NR. Adjuvant activity of a novel metabolizable lipid emulsion with inactivated viral vaccines. Infect Immun 1980; 28(3): 937–943.

Rice CM, Lenches EM, Eddy SR, Shin SJ, Sheets RL, Strauss JH. Nucleotide sequence of yellow fever virus: implications for flavivirus gene expression and evolution. Science 1985; 229(4715): 726–733.

Richman DD, Cleveland PH, McCormick JB, Johnson KM. Antigenic analysis of strains of Ebola virus: identification of two Ebola virus serotypes. J Infect Dis 1983; 147(2): 268–271.

Rico-Hesse R, Harrison LM, Salas RA, Tovar D, Nisalak A, Ramos C, Boshell J, de Mesa MT, Nogueira RM, da Rosa AT. Origins of dengue type 2 viruses associated with increased pathogenicity in the Americas. Virology 1997; 230(2): 244–251.

Rico-Hesse R, Harrison LM, Nisalak A, Vaughn DW, Kalayanarooj S, Green S, Rothman AL, Ennis FA. Molecular evolution of dengue type 2 virus in Thailand. Am J Trop Med Hyg 1998; 58(1): 96–101.

Rimoldi MT, de Bracco MM. In vitro inactivation of complement by a serum factor present in Junin-virus infected guinea-pigs. Immunology 1980; 39(2): 159–164.

Robert E, Vial T, Schaefer C, Arnon J, Reuvers M. Exposure to yellow fever vaccine in early pregnancy. Vaccine 1999; 17(3): 283–285.

Rodhain F. The role of monkeys in the biology of dengue and yellow fever. Comp Immunol Microbiol Infect Dis 1991; 14(1): 9–19.

Rodriguez LL, Maupin GO, Ksiazek TG, Rollin PE, Khan AS, Schwarz TF, Lofts RS, Smith JF, Noor AM, Peters CJ, Nichol ST. Molecular investigation of a multisource outbreak of Crimean-Congo hemorrhagic fever in the United Arab Emirates. Am J Trop Med Hyg 1997; 57(5): 512–518.

Rollin PE, Ksiazek TG, Jahrling PB, Haines M, Peters CJ. Detection of Ebola-like viruses by immunofluorescence. Lancet 1990; 336(8730): 1591.

Rothman AL, Kanesa-Thasan N, West K, Janus J, Saluzzo JF, Ennis FA. Induction of T lymphocyte responses to dengue virus by a candidate tetravalent live attenuated dengue virus vaccine. Vaccine 2001; 19(32): 4694–4699.

Rowe WP. Studies on Pathogenesis and Immunity in Lymphocytic Choriomeningitis Virus of the Mouse. Washington, DC: US Naval Medical Research Institute, Department of Defense; 1954 nm 005.048.14.01.

Ruigrok RW, Schoehn G, Dessen A, Forest E, Volchkov V, Dolnik O, Klenk HD, Weissenhorn W. Structural characterization and membrane binding properties of the matrix protein VP40 of Ebola virus. J Mol Biol 2000; 300(1): 103–112.

Russell PK, Nisalak A. Dengue virus identification by the plaque reduction neutralization test. J Immunol 1967; 99(2): 291–296.

Salas R, Manzione W, de Tesh RB, Rico-Hesse R, Shope RE, Betancourt A, Godoy O, Bruzual R, Pacheco ME, Ramos B, Taibo ME, Tamayo JG, Jaimes E, Vasquez C, Araoz F, Querales J. Venezuelan haemorrhagic fever. Lancet 1991; 338: 1033–1036.

Salas-Benito JS, del Angel RM. Identification of two surface proteins from C6/36 cells that bind dengue type 4 virus. J Virol 1997; 71(10): 7246–7252.

Salvato MS, Shimomaye EM. The completed sequence of lymphocytic choriomeningitis virus reveals a unique RNA structure and a gene for a zinc finger protein. Virology 1989; 173(1): 1–10.

Salvato MS, Schweighofer KJ, Burns J, Shimomaye EM. Biochemical and immunological evidence that the 11 kDa zinc-binding protein of lymphocytic choriomeningitis virus is a structural component of the virus. Virus Res 1992; 22(3): 185–198.

Sanchez A, Kiley MP. Identification and analysis of Ebola virus messenger RNA. Virology 1987; 157(2): 414–420.

Sanchez A, Trappier SG, Mahy BW, Peters CJ, Nichol ST. The virion glycoproteins of Ebola viruses are encoded in two reading frames and are expressed through transcriptional editing. Proc Natl Acad Sci USA 1996; 93(8): 3602–3607.

Sanchez A, Yang ZY, Xu L, Nabel GJ, Crews T, Peters CJ. Biochemical analysis of the secreted and virion glycoproteins of Ebola virus. J Virol 1998; 72(8): 6442–6447.

Sanchez AJ, Vincent MJ, Nichol ST. Characterization of the glycoproteins of Crimean-Congo hemorrhagic fever virus. J Virol 2002; 76(14): 7263–7275.

Schmaljohn CS. Bunyaviridae: the viruses and their replication. In: Fields Virology (Knipe D, Howley P, editors). 4th ed. Philadelphia: Lippincott, Williams & Wilkins; 2001; pp. 1581–1602.

Schmaljohn C, Hjelle B. Hantaviruses: a global disease problem. Emerg Infect Dis 1997; 3(2): 95–104.

Schmaljohn CS, Chu YK, Schmaljohn AL, Dalrymple JM. Antigenic subunits of Hantaan virus expressed by baculovirus and vaccinia virus recombinants. J Virol 1990; 64(7): 3162–3170.

Settergren B, Ahlm C, Juto P, Niklasson B. Specific Puumala IgG virus half a century after haemorrhagic fever with renal syndrome. Lancet 1991; 338(8758): 66.

Severson WE, Schmaljohn CS, Javadian A, Jonsson CB. Ribavirin causes error catastrophe during Hantaan virus replication. J Virol 2003; 77(1): 481–488.

Shurtleff AC, Beasley DW, Chen JJ, Ni H, Suderman MT, Wang H, Xu R, Wang E, Weaver SC, Watts DM, Russell KL, Barrett AD. Genetic variation in the $3'$ non-coding region of dengue viruses. Virology 2001; 281(1): 75–87.

Siam AL, Meegan JM, Gharbawi KF. Rift Valley fever ocular manifestations: observations during the 1977 epidemic in Egypt. Br J Ophthalmol 1980; 64(5): 366–374.

Simonetti SR, Schatzmayr HG, Barth OM, Simonetti JP. Detection of hepatitis B virus antigens in paraffin-embedded liver specimens from the Amazon region, Brazil. Mem Inst Oswaldo Cruz 2002; 97(1): 105–107.

Sjolander KB, Golovljova I, Vasilenko V, Plyusnin A, Lundkvist A. Serological divergence of Dobrava and Saaremaa hantaviruses: evidence for two distinct serotypes. Epidemiol Infect 2002; 128(1): 99–103.

Skehel JJ, Wiley DC. Coiled coils in both intracellular vesicle and viral membrane fusion. Cell 1998; 95(7): 871–874.

Smith GW, Wright PJ. Synthesis of proteins and glycoproteins in dengue type 2 virus-infected vero and *Aedes albopictus* cells. J Gen Virol 1985; 66(Pt 3): 559–571.

Song G, Huang YC, Hang CS, Hao FY, Li DX, Zheng XL, Liu WM, Li SL, Huo ZW, Huei LJ. Preliminary human trial of inactivated golden hamster kidney cell (GHKC) vaccine against haemorrhagic fever with renal syndrome (HFRS). Vaccine 1992; 10(4): 214–216.

Stephens HA, Klaythong R, Sirikong M, Vaughn DW, Green S, Kalayanarooj S, Endy TP, Libraty DH, Nisalak A, Innis BL, Rothman AL, Ennis FA, Chandanayingyong D. HLA-A and -B allele associations with secondary dengue virus infections correlate with disease severity and the infecting viral serotype in ethnic Thais. Tissue Antigens 2002; 60(4): 309–318.

Stephenson EH, Larson EW, Dominik JW. Effect of environmental factors on aerosol-induced Lassa virus infection. J Med Virol 1984; 14(4): 295–303.

Stephensen CB, Jacob JR, Montali RJ, Holmes KV, Muchmore E, Compans RW, Arms ED, Buchmeier MJ, Lanford RE. Isolation of an arenavirus from a marmoset with callitrichid hepatitis and its serologic association with disease. J Virol 1991; 65(8): 3995–4000.

Sullivan NJ, Sanchez A, Rollin PE, Yang ZY, Nabel GJ. Development of a preventive vaccine for Ebola virus infection in primates. Nature 2000; 408(6812): 605–609.

Sullivan NJ, Geisbert TW, Geisbert JB, Xu L, Yang ZY, Roederer M, et al. Accelerated vaccination for Ebola virus haemorrhagic fever in non-human primates. Nature 2003; 424(6949): 681–684.

Suzuki Y, Gojobori T. The origin and evolution of Ebola and Marburg viruses. Mol Biol Evol 1997; 14(8): 800–806.

Swanepoel R. Bunyaviridae. In: Principles and Practice of Clinical Virology (Zuckerman AJ, Banatvala JE, Pattison JR, editors). 4th ed. Chichester: Wiley; 2000; pp. 515–549.

Takada A, Kawaoka Y. The pathogenesis of Ebola hemorrhagic fever. Trends Microbiol 2001; 9(10): 506–511.

Takada A, Feldmann H, Stroeher U, Bray M, Watanabe S, Ito H, McGregor M, Kawaoka Y. Identification of protective epitopes on Ebola virus glycoprotein at the single amino acid level by using recombinant vesicular stomatitis viruses. J Virol 2003; 77(2): 1069–1074.

Tamura M, Asada H, Kondo K, Takahashi M, Yamanishi K. Effects of human and murine interferons against hemorrhagic fever with renal syndrome (HFRS) virus (Hantaan virus). Antivir Res 1987; 8(4): 171–178.

Tassaneetrithep B, Burgess TH, Granelli-Piperno A, Trumpfheller C, Finke J, Sun W, Eller MA, Pattanapanyasat K, Sarasombath S, Birx DL, Steinman RM, Schlesinger S, Marovich MA. DC-SIGN (CD209) mediates dengue virus infection of human dendritic cells. J Exp Med 2003; 197(7): 823–829.

Temonen M, Lankinen H, Vapalahti O, Ronni T, Julkunen I, Vaheri A. Effect of interferon-alpha and cell differentiation on Puumala virus infection in human monocyte/macrophages. Virology 1995; 206(1): 8–15.

Temonen M, Mustonen J, Helin H, Pasternack A, Vaheri A, Holthofer H. Cytokines, adhesion molecules, and cellular infiltration in nephropathia epidemica kidneys: an immunohistochemical study. Clin Immunol Immunopathol 1996; 78(1): 47–55.

Tesh RB, Jahrling PB, Salas R, Shope RE. Description of Guanarito virus (Arenaviridae: Arenavirus), the etiologic agent of Venezuelan hemorrhagic fever. Am J Trop Med Hyg 1994; 50(4): 452–459.

Timmins J, Schoehn G, Ricard-Blum S, Scianimanico S, Vernet T, Ruigrok RW, Weissenhorn W. Ebola virus matrix protein VP40 interaction with human cellular factors Tsg101 and Nedd4. J Mol Biol 2003; 326(2): 493–502.

Uzcategui NY, Camacho D, Comach G, Cuello dU, Holmes EC, Gould EA. Molecular epidemiology of dengue type 2 virus in Venezuela: evidence for in situ virus evolution and recombination. J Gen Virol 2001; 82(Pt 12): 2945–2953.

Van Epps HL, Schmaljohn CS, Ennis FA. Human memory cytotoxic T-lymphocyte (CTL) responses to Hantaan virus infection: identification of virus-specific and cross-reactive CD8(+) CTL epitopes on nucleocapsid protein. J Virol 1999; 73(7): 5301–5308.

Van Epps HL, Terajima M, Mustonen J, Arstila TP, Corey EA, Vaheri A, Ennis FA. Long-lived memory T lymphocyte responses after hantavirus infection. J Exp Med 2002; 196(5): 579–588.

Van Loock F, Thomas I, Clement J, Ghoos S, Colson P. A case-control study after a hantavirus infection outbreak in the south of Belgium: who is at risk? Clin Infect Dis 1999; 28(4): 834–839.

Vapalahti K, Paunio M, Brummer-Korvenkontio M, Vaheri A, Vapalahti O. Puumala virus infections in Finland: increased occupational risk for farmers. Am J Epidemiol 1999a; 149(12): 1142–1151.

Vapalahti O, Lundkvist A, Fedorov V, Conroy CJ, Hirvonen S, Plyusnina A, Nemirov K, Fredga K, Cook JA, Niemimaa J, Kaikusalo A, Henttonen H, Vaheri A, Plyusnin A. Isolation and characterization of a hantavirus from *Lemmus sibiricus*: evidence for host switch during hantavirus evolution. J Virol 1999; 73(7): 5586–5592.

Vapalahti O, Mustonen J, Lundkvist A, Henttonen H, Plyusnin A, Vaheri A. Hantavirus infections in Europe. Lancet Infect Dis 2003; 3(10): 653–661.

Vaughn DW, Green S, Kalayanarooj S, Innis BL, Nimmannitya S, Suntayakorn S, Endy TP, Raengsakulrach B, Rothman AL, Ennis FA, Nisalak A. Dengue viremia titer, antibody response pattern, and virus serotype correlate with disease severity. J Infect Dis 2000; 181(1): 2–9.

Volchkov VE, Blinov VM, Netesov SV. The envelope glycoprotein of Ebola virus contains an immunosuppressive-like domain similar to oncogenic retroviruses. FEBS Lett 1992; 305(3): 181–184.

Volchkov VE, Chepurnov AA, Volchkova VA, Ternovoj VA, Klenk HD. Molecular characterization of guinea pig-adapted variants of Ebola virus. Virology 2000; 277(1): 147–155.

Volchkov VE, Volchkova VA, Muhlberger E, Kolesnikova LV, Weik M, Dolnik O, Klenk HD. Recovery of infectious Ebola virus from complementary DNA: RNA editing of the GP gene and viral cytotoxicity. Science 2001; 291(5510): 1965–1969.

Walker DH, Murphy FA. Pathology and pathogenesis of arenavirus infections. Curr Top Microbiol Immunol 1987; 133: 89–113.

Wang E, Ryman KD, Jennings AD, Wood DJ, Taffs F, Minor PD, Sanders PG, Barrett AD. Comparison of the genomes of the wild-type French viscerotropic strain of yellow fever virus with its vaccine derivative French neurotropic vaccine. J Gen Virol 1995; 76(Pt 11): 2749–2755.

Wang E, Ni H, Xu R, Barrett AD, Watowich SJ, Gubler DJ, Weaver SC. Evolutionary relationships of endemic/epidemic and sylvatic dengue viruses. J Virol 2000; 74(7): 3227–3234.

Watts DM, Porter KR, Putvatana P, Vasquez B, Calampa C, Hayes CG, Halstead SB. Failure of secondary infection with American genotype dengue 2 to cause dengue haemorrhagic fever. Lancet 1999; 354(9188): 1431–1434.

Weissenhorn W, Calder LJ, Wharton SA, Skehel JJ, Wiley DC. The central structural feature of the membrane fusion protein subunit from the Ebola virus glycoprotein is a long triple-stranded coiled coil. Proc Natl Acad Sci USA 1998; 95(11): 6032–6036.

Whitton JL, Gebhard JR, Lewicki H, Tishon A, Oldstone MBA. Molecular definition of a major cytotoxic T-lymphocyte epitope in the glycoprotein of lymphocytic choriomeningitis virus. J Virol 1988; 62(3): 687–695.

Wilson JA, Hart MK. Protection from Ebola virus mediated by cytotoxic T lymphocytes specific for the viral nucleoprotein. J Virol 2001; 75(6): 2660–2664.

Wilson JA, Hevey M, Bakken R, Guest S, Bray M, Schmaljohn AL, Hart MK. Epitopes involved in antibody-mediated protection from Ebola virus. Science 2000; 287(5458): 1664–1666.

Woodruff AW. Handling patients with suspected Lassa fever entering Great Britain. Bull World Health Organ 1975; 52(4–6): 717–721.

Wu SJ, Grouard-Vogel G, Sun W, Mascola JR, Brachtel E, Putvatana R, Louder MK, Filgueira L, Marovich MA, Wong HK, Blauvelt A, Murphy GS, Robb ML, Innes BL, Birx DL, Hayes CG, Frankel SS. Human skin Langerhans cells are targets of dengue virus infection. Nat Med 2000; 6(7): 816–820.

Wylie JAH, Collier LH. The English sweating sickness (Sudor Anglicus): a reappraisal. J Med Hist 1981; 36: 425–445.

Xu L, Sanchez A, Yang Z, Zaki SR, Nabel EG, Nichol ST, Nabel GJ. Immunisation for Ebola virus infection. Nat Med 1998; 4: 37–42.

Yadani FZ, Kohl A, Prehaud C, Billecocq A, Bouloy M. The carboxy-terminal acidic domain of Rift Valley Fever virus NSs protein is essential for the formation of filamentous structures but not for the nuclear localization of the protein. J Virol 1999; 73(6): 5018–5025.

Yamanishi K, Tanishita O, Tamura M, Asada H, Kondo K, Takagi M, Yoshida I, Konobe T, Fukai K. Development of inactivated vaccine against virus causing haemorrhagic fever with renal syndrome. Vaccine 1988; 6(3): 278–282.

Yang Z-Y, Delgado R, Xu L, Todd RF, Nabel EG, Sanchez A, Nabel GJ. Distinct cellular interactions of secreted and transmembrane Ebola virus glycoproteins. Science 1998; 279: 1034–1037.

Yang ZY, Duckers HJ, Sullivan NJ, Sanchez A, Nabel EG, Nabel GJ. Identification of the Ebola virus glycoprotein as the main viral determinant of vascular cell cytotoxicity and injury. Nat Med 2000; 6(8): 886–889.

Yedloutschnig RJ, Dardiri AH, Walker JS, Peters CJ, Eddy GA. Immune response of steers, goats and sheep to inactivated Rift Valley Fever vaccine. Proc Annu Meet US Anim Health Assoc 1979; 83: 253–260.

Yen YC, Kong LX, Lee L, Zhang YQ, Li F, Cai BJ, et al. Characteristics of Crimean-Congo hemorrhagic fever virus (Xinjiang strain) in China. Am J Trop Med Hyg 1985; 34(6): 1179–1182.

Young PR. Arenaviridae. In: Animal Virus Structures (Nermut MV, Steven AC, editors). Amsterdam: Elsevier; 1987; pp. 185–198.

Young PR, Howard CR. Fine structure analysis of Pichinde virus nucleocapsids. J Gen Virol 1983; 64(Pt 4): 833–842.

Zaki AM. Isolation of a flavivirus related to the tick-borne encephalitis complex from human cases in Saudi Arabia. Trans R Soc Trop Med Hyg 1997; 91(2): 179–181.

Zaki SR, Greer PW, Coffield LM, Goldsmith CS, Nolte KB, Foucar K, Feddersen RM, Zumwalt RE, Miller GL, Khan AS. Hantavirus pulmonary syndrome. Pathogenesis of an emerging infectious disease. Am J Pathol 1995; 146(3): 552–579.

Zaki SR, Shieh WJ, Greer PW, Goldsmith CS, Ferebee T, Katshitshi J, Tshioko FK, Bwaka MA, Swanepoel R, Calain P, Khan AS, Lloyd E, Rollin PE, Ksiazek TG, Peters CJ. A novel immunohistochemical assay for the detection of Ebola virus in skin: implications for diagnosis, spread, and surveillance of Ebola hemorrhagic fever. Commission de Lutte contre les Epidemies a Kikwit. J Infect Dis 1999; 179(Suppl 1): S36–S47.

Zanotto PM, Gould EA, Gao GF, Harvey PH, Holmes EC. Population dynamics of flaviviruses revealed by molecular phylogenies. Proc Natl Acad Sci USA 1996; 93(2): 548–553.

Zeitz PS, Butler JC, Cheek JE, Samuel MC, Childs JE, Shands LA, Turner RE, Voorhees RE, Sarisky J, Rollin PE. A case-control study of hantavirus pulmonary syndrome during an outbreak in the southwestern United States. J Infect Dis 1995; 171(4): 864–870.

Zeitz PS, Graber JM, Voorhees RA, Kioski C, Shands LA, Ksiazek TG, Jenison S, Khabbaz RF. Assessment of occupational risk for hantavirus infection in Arizona and New Mexico. J Occup Environ Med 1997; 39(5): 463–467.

Zhu ZY, Tang HY, Li YJ, Weng JQ, Yu YX, Zeng RF. Investigation on inactivated epidemic hemorrhagic fever tissue culture vaccine in humans. Chin Med J (Engl) 1994; 107(3): 167–170.

Zinkernagel RM, Doherty PC. MHC-restricted cytotoxic T-cells: studies on the biological role of polymorphic major transplantation antigens determining T-cell restriction-specificity, function and responsiveness. Adv Immunol 1979; 27: 151–177.

Index